Homoeopathy For Farm And Garden

Toward A Homoeopathic Agriculture

VAIKUNTHANATH DAS KAVIRAJ

"A crank is a man with a new idea - until it catches on ..." M Twain

Mark Moodie Publications. Oaklands Park, Newnham-on-Severn, Gloucester, GL14 1EF, UK
http://www.moodie.biz

ISBN-10; 0-9517890-5-8
ISBN-13; 978-0-9517890-5-6
EAN; 9780951789056

Contents

Materia Medica 42

Homoeopathic Foundation

The scientific foundation of this book is classical homoeopathy. For the majority of modern people this will necessitate a change of perspective; instead of focusing our efforts on the pest or disease, it is the plant that suffers and, therefore, the plant that should be the centre of investigation.

In 'chemical agriculture', massive doses of highly toxic substances are applied to combat pests or disease symptoms directly. Hahnemann[1] says about such practice: "In estimating the value of this mode of employing medicines, we should even pass over the circumstance that it is an extremely faulty symptomatic treatment, wherein the practitioner devotes his attention in a merely one-sided manner to a single symptom, consequently to only a small part of the whole, whereby relief for the totality of disease, cannot evidently be expected." (Organon #58.)

And further: "Had physicians been capable of reflection on the sad results of the antagonistic employment of medicines, they had long since discovered the grand truth, THAT THE TRUE RADICAL HEALING ART MUST BE FOUND IN THE EXACT OPPOSITE OF SUCH AN ANTIPATHIC TREATMENT OF THE SYMPTOMS OF DISEASE." (Organon #61.)

Hahnemann asserts that there is only temporary relief in treatment that deals with only one symptom. Observation of modern agricultural practice reveals that this antipathic treatment is the order of the day. The amount of chemicals used is awesome and the buildup of resistance among the diseases and pests is one of the consequences. Considering the prevalent ideas within agricultural science, one can see that if it is not entirely faulty, it is at least not entirely rational.

Kent says in his 'Philosophy': "We daily see that the antipathic and heteropathic methods have no permanence. By these means there are effected changes in the economy and changes in the symptoms but no permanent cure, the tendency being simply to the establishment of another disease, often worse than the first and without eradicating the first." (Lectures on The Philosophy, page 90.)

The Cause of Disease

"Therefore disease, considered as a thing separate from the living whole, from the organism and its animating vital force and hidden in the interior, be it of ever so subtle a character, is an absurdity that could only be imagined by minds of the

1 - Samuel Hahnemann 1755 - 1843. Founder of homoeopathy. His central text is the 'Organon'.

materialistic stamp." (Organon #13.) And further: "The natural disease is never to be considered as a noxious material situated somewhere in the exterior or interior." (Organon #148.)

Susceptibility to pests and disease is caused by the stress induced by wrong spacing, cultivation, artificial fertilisers, and chemicals to control pests or diseases. From the effects of these chemicals we could learn more about the treatment for plants.

"... diseases are nothing more than alterations in the state of health of the individual, which express themselves by morbid signs." (Organon #19.) As in humans who suffer from parasitical worms, scabies, lice, fleas and other pests which sometimes carry deadly diseases such as yellow fever, so too in plants we see the same; aphids carry yellow dwarf virus, and there are a host of pests besides the aphid that can disturb the life of plants profoundly.

Besides this there are the massive doses of fertiliser, herbicides, pesticides and fungicides, each of which will influence the plant to show more or less how they are affected through signs and symptoms. Considering the effects of agricultural chemicals we must keep in mind the following: ".... Medicines could never cure diseases if they did not have the power of altering the state of health ... their curative power must be owing solely to this power they possess of altering the state of health." (Organon #19.)

Thus Kent says: "We know very well that in the old school [i.e. the chemical school in agriculture], there is no plan laid down for acquiring a knowledge of medicines except by experimenting with them on the sick. Hahnemann condemns this as dangerous because it subjects the sufferers to hardship, and because of its uncertainty." (Lectures on The Philosophy, page 170.)

When we apply this approach to plants and how they thrive in nature or in the sensible cultivation of food plants, we note, for instance, that companion plants exist in great variety. Only a few of them have been included in this book, mainly due to insufficient availability of plants upon which to test them. The warnings about growing too many companion plants with a crop are a warning of a sort of 'proving'[2]. The reports of excess and deficiency of nutrients can also be seen as crude provings. Hahnemann has the following to say about this: "Much more frequent than the natural diseases associating with and complicating one another in the same body, are the morbid complications which the inappropriate treatment is apt to produce by the long continued employment of unsuitable drugs." (Organon #41.)

We are led to believe that chemical treatment is harmless to the plant, notwithstanding a withholding period imposed on crops that have been sprayed. The reason given

---

2 - A 'proving' is an experiment to see what symptoms are evoked in healthy subjects by a substance. Since 'like cures like', these are the same symptoms addressed by a homoeopathic remedy.

is that the poisons can break down or wash off in this time, as it is considered dangerous for people to consume freshly sprayed produce. The assertion that it is safe for the plants is, in this light, a questionable conclusion.

"Every agent that acts upon the vitality, every medicine, deranges more or less the vital force and causes a certain alteration in the health of the individual for a shorter or longer period." (Organon #63.)

Applied to the life of plants, this includes the use of herbicides, pesticides, fungicides and chemical fertilisers. Examples of this will be found throughout this book.

"Every real medicine acts at all times, under all circumstances, on every living being and produces its peculiar symptoms, distinctly perceptible if the dose be large enough. (Organon #32.)

'Because sugar is not arsenic many graves are full'. From the reports written on the effects of these substances on plants much information can be found as to the abuse of this method of feeding and treating plant pests and diseases. They furnish the rudimentary outline of this materia medica. "...it was never suspected that these histories of medicinal diseases would furnish the first rudiments of the true pure materia medica, which has until now consisted solely on false conjectures and fictions of the imagination." (Organon #110.) "Medicinal substances act in the morbid changes they produce according to fixed eternal laws of nature to produce certain reliable disease symptoms, each according to its own peculiar character." (Organon #111.)

The Totality of Symptoms

"Useful to the physician in assisting him to cure are the particulars of the most probable exciting cause ... In these investigations the ascertainable physical constitution, ... mode of living and habitat ... age and sexual function are to be taken into consideration." (Organon #5.)

Kent gives us the following description of the totality of symptoms: "The 'totality of symptoms' means a good deal. It may be considered to be all that is essential to the disease. It is all that is apparent and represents the disease in the natural world to the eye, the touch and external understanding of man." ('Lectures on The Philosophy', page 85.)

More attention must be given to the plant and its habitat, particularly with pot-plants. The type of soil, the relative size of the pot and the plant, the proximity of inimical plants, its position in regards to light and any other factors that may influence the action of a remedy must be considered. This is not to say that these factors should in any way be neglected in the free standing plants. As we shall see, it appears that in pot plants this is of greater significance.

"The unprejudiced observer, be his powers of penetration ever so great, takes note of nothing in every individual case, except the changes in the health of the body which he can perceive externally by means of the senses." (Organon #6.) These changes may include plant pathology reports, chemical analysis and microscopic evidence. As plants do not readily communicate their state of health other than through visible symptoms, these pathology reports are often necessary to complement the visible signs and arrive at the totality of symptoms.

"Now, as in a disease … we can perceive nothing but the morbid symptoms, it must be the symptoms alone by which the disease demands and points to the remedy suited to remove it – and, moreover, the totality of these symptoms ... must be the principal, indeed the only thing the physician has to take note of in every case of disease ..." (Organon #7.) "… after removal of all the symptoms of the disease and of the entire collection of the perceptible phenomena there should or could remain anything else besides health ..." (Organon #8.) "… besides the totality of symptoms, with consideration of the accompanying modalities nothing can be discovered." (Organon #18.)

There is no relevance in anything else. Hahnemann concludes: "... that the sum of all the symptoms and conditions in each individual case of disease must be the sole indication, the sole guide to direct us in the choice of a remedy." (Organon #18.) "…if the patient complain of a few violent sufferings, … on investigation several other symptoms will be found besides, which furnish a complete picture of the disease." (Organon #151.)

By extension from human suffering to that of plants, this suggests the usefulness of plant pathology reports, in which the chemical analysis, microscopic evidence and other relevant signs and symptoms such as soil nutrient levels, will add to the picture of the disease. For instance, excess levels of certain nutrients can trigger pest population explosions, while some pests are vectors for plant diseases.

The Similimum

I trust that it is evident from these paragraphs that for plants too, the totality of symptoms is the only means by which they can be successfully treated. Therefore, the necessity of finding the correct remedy has to be assessed in order to cure the plant permanently. "… it follows, on the one hand, that medicines only become remedies and capable of annihilating diseases, because the medicinal substance, by exciting certain effects and symptoms … removes and abrogates the symptoms already present." (Organon #22.)

These paragraphs indicate that the records and comments here produced as regards the action on plants are not based on conjecture, but on sound scientific principles. This is because; "Neither in the course of nature, nor by the physician's art, can an existing affection or malady in any one instance be removed by a dissimilar agent ...

but solely by one that is similar in symptoms ... according to eternal irrevocable laws of nature." (Organon, #48.)

The oldest reference to the 'Law of Similars' (which Hahnemann traced back as far as Hippocrates, who derived the idea from the Arab physicians, who in turn took it from Vedic India) is found in the Bhagavat Purana, which was written 5,000 years ago. There it literally says:

"O good soul, does not a thing, when applied therapeutically, cure a disease which was caused by that very same thing?"
(SB 1-5-33)

"There are but two principal methods of cure: the one based only on accurate observation of nature, on careful experimentation and pure experience, the homoeopathic, and a second which does not do this, the heteropathic or allopathic." (Organon #52.)

"A third mode of employing medicines in diseases has been attempted to be created by means of 'isopathy', as it is called – that is to say, a method of curing a given disease by the same contagious principle that produces it." (Organon #56, footnote.) Hahnemann says that this is not really the same, because it is given in a potentised form, thus having been altered to a similimum. Hahnemann always stresses the totality of symptoms and in likewise manner proceeds to inform us that the similimum is the only remedy specific to the case before us.

He further says: "The curative power of medicines, therefore, depends on their symptoms, similar to the disease ... so that each individual case of disease is most surely, radically, rapidly, and permanently annihilated and removed only by a medicine capable of producing in the most similar and complete manner, the totality of its symptoms." (Organon #27.)

Kent elaborates on this in the following manner: "Then it is not sufficient merely to give the drug itself, regardless of its form. It is not sufficient to give the crude drug, but the plane upon which it is to be given is a question of study. In a proving, the crude drug may bring forth a mass of symptoms in one prover, but when a person is sick those symptoms will not be touched by the crude drug." (Lectures on The Philosophy, page 93.)

That this is no mere theory has been borne out by countless experiments: "As this natural law of cure manifests itself in every pure experiment and every true observation in the world, the fact is consequently established; it matters little what may be the scientific explanation of how it takes place." (Organon, #28.)

The Single Remedy

There is another important point in the treatment of plants which I feel should be given the utmost attention, since it is often neglected in the treatment of humans even among the homoeopathic fraternity. This is the absolute necessity of the administration of the single remedy.

"In no case under treatment is it necessary and, therefore, permissible to administer to a patient more than one single simple medicinal substance at one time. It is **absolutely not allowed** in homoeopathy." (Organon, #273.) Hahnemann also says: "It is wrong to attempt to employ complex means when simple means suffice." (Organon, #274.)

The Minimum Dose

As plants are sensitive living beings, the necessity of using the minimum dose, also often neglected in the treatment of people, cannot be stressed enough. As the power of a medicine increases with the reduction in quantity when prepared according to the homoeopathic method, it follows that the quantity given must diminish in proportion to the increase in potency. Because plants, with obvious exceptions, have much smaller bodies than humans it follows that the dose administered should be the smallest possible. Hahnemann says this about it.: "If we give too strong a dose of a medicine … it must … prove injurious by its mere magnitude." (Organon, #275.)

And further: "… a medicine … does harm in every dose that is too large … In strong doses it does more harm the greater its homoeopathicity and the higher the potency selected. Too large doses … especially when frequently repeated, bring about much trouble as a rule. (Organon, #276.)

Routinely prescribing repetitive doses is poor practice. Hahnemann continues: "They put the patient not seldom in danger of life or make his disease almost incurable." (Organon, #276.)

Hahnemann further warns against repetition of the dose in the 'Chronic Diseases', where he states: "(Medicines) ... given in the most appropriate dose, are the less effective the oftener they were repeated. They served at last hardly even as weak palliatives." (Chronic Diseases, pg 3 & 4.)

Even with the highest potencies he does not condone repeated doses unconditionally, as we can see in the Organon where he describes the possibilities of the LM potencies: "The same carefully selected medicine **may** now be given daily and for months **if necessary** in this way … (Organon, #246 footnote 185. Emphasis mine.)

The words 'may' and 'if necessary' are the operative words here and practitioners would do well to take heed, especially in plants.

Von Boenninghausen says: "For a scientific establishment of the curative power and efficiency of the high potencies, we cite the well-established law of nature discovered by Maupertuis and mathematically proved by him. This we apply to therapy. This is the law of the least effects, by others called the '*Lex parsimoniae*'. The discoverer stated it in the following words: '*La quantite d'action necessaire pour causer quelque changement dans la nature, est la plus petite qu'il soit possible*,' i.e. the quantity of action necessary to produce any change in nature, is the smallest that is possible." (Von Boenninghausen, The Lesser Writings, page 146.) Hahnemann said that it is folly to use large means where small means suffice. "This law of effects (minimus maxima) appears, therefore, to be an essential and necessary complement to the law of homoeopathy (similia similibus) and to occupy a similar place with it." (Von Boenninghausen, The Lesser Writings, page 147.)

Von Boenninghausen quotes Hahnemann's 'Chronic Diseases' in his 'Lesser Writings' in the following passage: "If ... the medicines do not act out their full time while they are still acting, the whole cure will amount to nothing." (Chronic Diseases, page 124.)

"The fundamental rule in this respect remains," so says Von Boenninghausen – and then quotes Hahnemann again: "To allow the dose of the medicine selected ... to complete its action undisturbed, so long as it visibly furthers the cure, ... a process which forbids every new prescription ... <u>as also the repetition of the same remedy</u>." (Chronic Diseases, pages 124-125.)

I do not think that further quotes are necessary to impress upon the reader the necessity of the single dose in plants, as even in ourselves this is plainly obvious from the writings of the old masters. Having established the rules that govern the use of homoeopathy in plants – based on the same natural laws that govern its use in humans and animals – I will conclude this foundation with a few remarks about the work so far conducted.

The remedies made from insect pests do not always work equally well and, as a consequence, are not easy to prescribe. Some remedies, such as aphid, did not produce any results either from trituration or solution. This may be due to the method of preparation – some have been triturated, some exist in dilution. They appear to have different action between trituration and dilution but this may also be due to the method used in their application. But as not all methods of preparation have been exhausted, there may be a reaction from *Aphis tosta*, which is one remedy that will be produced in this manner in the near future.

Experiments were often conducted by those not familiar with homoeopathy but from the mistakes resulting from this, at times, exciting new phenomena were discovered. These are described with some of the remedies. Some were used repeatedly because of re-infestation and this may have caused a form of proving. Especially in pot-plants this re-infestation was marked. This might be due to the fact that free standing plants take up the remedy only for a short period, while the water in which they have been suspended leaches through the soil. In pot-plants, this water collects at the bottom of the pot, which allows the plant much longer exposure to the remedy, taking up a much larger dose. The concept of the minimum dose is thus violated with the result that a proving is instigated. Rather than discouraging, these incidents point to the necessity of repeated experiments with different plants and remedies, preferably under different circumstances. It also points to the necessity of provings which I have not been able to conduct. It is, after all, a bit much to ask friends or commercial growers to part with the results of many hours of hard work, merely to satisfy the curiosity of a homoeopath.

Although in homoeopathy we do not use complexes, interesting experiments can be instigated where some of these remedies can be mixed in the crude, from which combination a tincture can be prepared. This is a similar to the process of production of a remedy, which is mixed in the crude after which the potencies are made, for example *Hepar sulphate calcarea* and others. These are not complexes but simplexes.

It is evident that I have, so far, only scratched the surface. Nonetheless I see a great future ahead for both homoeopathy and agriculture. Homoeopathy will be given more credibility as a scientific method and agriculture will be enriched with cleaner control measures. This will also be beneficial to the environment. The charges laid at our door concerning the placebo effect can also no longer be upheld. Although this was already clearly demonstrated with animals, this will constitute further proof that these charges are baseless. Besides, many experiments have been conducted to prove the existence of something in our potencies, of which I will give some examples here.

- In 1948 Wormer and Loch tested several substances from 24x to 30x. They used a photoelectric cell to measure the intensity and wavelength of these potencies and found measurable changes, of both intensity and wavelength in these substances.
- In the years 1951-3, Gay and Boiron tested both distilled water, and *Natrum muriaticum* in the 27c potency for their dielectric constant. They were able to show that the potency of *Natrum muriaticum* could be easily selected from among 99 control bottles.
- Boericke and Smith, in 1963 tested a 12x potency of *Sulphur*, with and without succussion. They tested the solvent structure by nuclear magnetic resonance spectrum. They found that there were structural changes in the solvent as the potency was increased by succussion, while no such change was detected in the controls.
- Stephenson and Brucato in 1966 tested both distilled water and *Merc.cor.* from the 1x to the 33x. They found that the dielectric constant for the controls varied from 5.6 to 6.05. For the homoeopathic potencies it varied from 2.8 to 4.4.
- Young in 1975 tested *Sulphur* from 5x to 30x, with controls. He also tested the solvent structure by nuclear magnetic resonance spectrum. He found that there were measurable changes in the spectra at each dilution and succussion. No such changes were observed for the solution without succussion or without *Sulphur*.

• In 1976, Boiron and Vinh used Raman Laser Spectroscopy, showing that for the 1c potency of *Kali bichromicum* the spectrum of alcohol disappears completely, while that for potassium bichromate appears. In *Kali bich.* 1c the ratio of the number of potassium bichromate molecules is 1 to 500. In such a case the light meets 500 more alcohol molecules as those of bichromate, yet the alcohol spectrum does not appear.
• In 1982, Resch, Gutman and Schauer found that dilute sodium chloride solutions revealed an increase in electrical conductivity, by rocking them prior to measurement.
• Four French researchers developed a method of detection through nuclear magnetic resonance, conducted in the late 80's, which shows specific waves for each potency, as well as a specific wave for the substance used. These latter remain the same throughout all potencies of that substance, while the wave expressing the potencies are specific to those potencies. Thus a clear and recognisable scientifically provable frame of reference exists, for each remedy and potency.

From these examples it is obvious that there exist a particular quality in homoeopathic medicine even beyond Avogadro's limit, not found in dilutions. I mention this because I expect some resistance from the mechanistic heads at work in the diverse agricultural research facilities who will, no doubt, put forward many objections against the use of homoeopathy on plants.

This field of work deserves, however, to be explored to its limits and I hope that I have aroused sufficient curiosity in my colleagues for them to contribute to its expansion.

Finally, I apologise for any discrepancies or errors which may have crept in, notwithstanding scrupulous editing. I express the hope that it may serve the homoeopathic fraternity and all those interested in growing plants, whether for pleasure or for a living, in the manner intended.

Agriculture

Long before anybody used modern agricultural methods, farmers used to grow crops using simple methods.

They used manure for the soil and herbal sprays when pests or diseases attacked the plants. They used companion plants, such as chamomile, among the vegetables. Beans and corn, or basil and tomatoes have been grown together since Greek and Roman times.

Some very old practices which stood the test of time, are tree-flogging which dislodges hibernating insects, removes excess fruit spurs, releases sap, or splits bark and stimulates growth. This is still practised in many cultures. Baker asserts that it relates "to the innate relationship of humans to plants, rather than cross-cultural exchange." With the industrial revolution and the introduction of harvesting machinery, the monoculture made its appearance. From this time the farmers used sprays in large amounts and insects gradually became resistant.

The first pest and disease control measures were aimed at a knock-out, non-selective elimination. Wood ash, soot, chalk, dust, tar, fumigation or ammonia were the not-always ecologically sound products, because both the predators and beneficial insects were killed. The use of acids, salts and soap was common. Herbals like tobacco, derris, rue, artemisia and others, as well as elemental copper, arsenic, lead, mercury and sulphur were lethal to insect populations. The latter group was detrimental not only to the insects, but also the environment and the people who consumed the crops.

Coal tar, extensively used at the early twentieth century, is a powerful insecticide. It was also used as wood preservative and herbicide. Mineral oils were used as winter washes, smothering and dispersing agents. They are used to this very day. Resistance to insecticides was recorded as early as 1945. (Conacher, 1979.)

The "Clean Foods Act" was introduced in the USA around this time, to set standards for acceptable chemical residues in food as a response to controversial levels of arsenic in fruit and lead in other crops.

In the 1930s Swiss researchers discovered the insecticidal properties of the organo-chlorines, originally synthesized in 1874. This resulted in DDT, extensively used during the last years of the World War II and only recently banned in most industrial nations.

In the 1950s the organochlorines Dieldrin and Aldrin, and the organo-phosphates Malathion and Diazion were developed. Carbamates like Ferbam, Zineb and Captan, the herbicides Diurin, Simazin, and Paraquat found their way to the market. Within a short period of time the effectiveness of these products diminished and, at the same time, they proved highly toxic to the environment.

The search was then directed to biological agents. Predatory mites were bred such as wasps against aphids, and microbial agents like Bacillus thuringiensis were developed. In Australia, the CSIRO in concert with the State Agricultural Departments introduced fungal diseases, such as rust fungi against weeds. Moths, beetles and parasitic wasps were used against insect pests. That this is not necessarily a happy practice is evident from the increase of fungal diseases in food crops. The best alternative was the use of pheromones of plants and insects as they have no side effects and no build-up of resistance.

All these programs and methods lose sight of the real problem - the fact that it is the plants which are still being attacked by pests and diseases. Trying to eradicate pests and diseases amounts to a wild goose chase because neither the pest nor the disease is the problem. The plant is having the problem so, therefore, the plant needs the treatment.

When a pest is sprayed, all it achieves is thinning the local pest population. This invites other members of the same species to fill the gap so little more than a delay in pest attack is achieved. Homoeopathic remedies treat the plant, not the pest or disease. This results in stronger healthy plants which are unacceptable to pests, and not prone to disease attack.

Inter-cropping with companion plants also deserves much more attention than it gets. Yet very few farmers use the companion plant method because harvesting machinery is not equipped for dual tasks. For monoculture farming the homoeopathic approach is the best possible answer.

Homoeopathic medicine applies remedies in doses that are much smaller than conventional and even biodynamic methods, so no harmful residual traces are introduced into the environment. Even highly toxic substances such as arsenic become virtually harmless in highly diluted form, whilst remaining effective in plants that suffer from pest or disease attack. Plants only absorb micro-doses of any substance, hence a homoeopathic remedy is particularly adapted for the treatment of plants. Both as a spray or in the trickle system, a remedy is absorbed in the shortest possible time. Both the leaves and the roots absorb a remedy well.

A plant is, to some extent, similar to a human body. Our mucous membranes are situated in the interior of the body while in a plant they are on the exterior, protected only by thin epidermis. Thus the lungs and digestive system form the leaves of the plant, the capillary system resembles human blood circulation, the urinary system is represented by evaporation through the leaves. Sugars and protein represent the fat reserves and the muscular tissue. When a plant is diseased or suffers from a pest attack, its sugar and protein levels are depleted in a similar manner to the fat and muscular tissues of the human body.

Natural agricultural practices prevent pests and diseases 90-95% of the time. In chemical agriculture such prevention is difficult. This book is written for homoeopaths and the farmers who are using chemicals but want an alternative.

What is presented here comes from my personal experience and that of my colleagues, from confirmed knowledge regarding the companion plants, from published information on agriculture, and from the homoeopathic materia medica in analogy with plants.

The Commercial Method

Just off USA highway 40 on the edge of a research park, sits a building of one of the world's biggest agrochemical producers. In the lobby a glass case rotates displaying a basket of plastic fruit and vegetables. A computer screen displays the weather and market information. The company motto on its brochures proudly proclaims, "Helping to feed the world". Of all the people in the building it is unlikely that a single one has ever set foot on a farm, let alone on a small plot in Asia, Africa or Latin America. This is the headquarters of Rhone-Poulenc, one of the biggest promoters of pesticides. It is poised on the edge of also becoming the biggest promoter of genetically engineered crops. Together with Calgene, they have engineered cotton so that it is now immune to the herbicide Bromoxynil. This is because this herbicide not only kills weeds, but the cotton as well. This amounts to good business because it helps the sale of Bromoxynil.

In 1993, Ciba-Geigy began an ambitious project to immunise plants. The idea is straightforward; plants, like animals and humans, have an immune system which can be stimulated to give plants resistance to diseases and pests. The world's farmers spend some US$25 billion on chemical pesticides each year. However, it is not as effective as the farmers would like it to be. Pests and diseases still take about 30% of the annual crops worldwide, of which 12% is through diseases and 18% from pests.

Unfortunately, immunising crops is not altogether problem-free. Sometimes it can inhibit plant growth, presumably because defence mechanisms divert food resources from a plant's growth mechanisms. Also, when employed too vigorously, defence mechanisms may damage the plant itself. Some of the substances made in response to diseases, are toxic both to the plant and the disease. Biologists have to overcome these 'side-effects' if they are to sell the idea to the farmers. Another problem encountered with transgenic implanted pest and disease resistance, is that a few generations later the pests and diseases have built up resistance and the farmer and his crop are back to square one.

Organic farmers, who are known for their anti-pesticide stance, do not welcome the new techniques all that enthusiastically. It is really answering the wrong question. Farmers are wary about the possible effects of immunization techniques and in particular of genetically engineered crops. It is producing seeds for a global monoculture.

The Natural Method

As far back as 1911 a landmark book was written by Franklin King; 'Farmers of Forty Centuries; Permanent Agriculture in China, Korea and Japan.' It describes how farmers in Asia have worked their fields for over 4,000 years, without depleting the fertility of the soil. This book, and others written at the beginning of the 20th century, focus on the holistic aspects of agriculture in which the farmer tries to imitate nature rather than fighting a losing battle against it. The holistic approach and the complete farming systems which require companion planting to make room for natural predators of crop pests, form the core of these books.

In the book 'Earthkeeping', Gordon Harrison states that: "Mature stable systems – those that have reached the so-called climax state of succession – are usually remarkably conservative of minerals. One ecologist calculated that a certain New Hampshire forest, using about 365 pounds of calcium per acre to nourish life within it, lost annually about 8 pounds per acre by run-off. Of this, 3 pounds was replaced by rain and the other 5 by fresh weathering of rock. Incidentally, it was observed that when trees were cut, vastly greater amounts of calcium washed away."

Elsewhere the author states: "Diversity is associated with stability, as both cause and effect. Redundancy in a system is the best insurance against break-down."

Spatial arrangements in nature prevent the crowding of any species. By growing single crops the farmer tries to out do natural arrangements. In nature, the available space tends to be occupied by as great a variety as the natural habitat allows. This is the mechanism by which nature eliminates disease and thus the extermination of any one species of plant or animal. Too many animals or plants of the same species in too little space, triggers a mechanism that either prevents breeding, or makes up for the excess through more rapid death.

All stable natural systems have these switches, but not all populations do. People, as noted, do not have any of these switches if the rate at which the global population expands is anything to go by. Pests, notably insects like the Colorado-beetle, the locust, and rodents like rats, have none. They are species whose populations are entirely regulated by outside forces, in relation to the availability of food. Pests of this kind produce far more offspring than is needed to keep the population stable, or that can be normally supported. A farmer planting a crop of their favourite food creates a situation that results in a massive reduction of the pests' infant mortality rate. It does not require any cynicism to see the parallel with man.

"The species that explodes its population is per definition a pest and the latest addition to the ever-growing list of injurious pests is, of course, man himself." (Harrison, 'Earthkeeping'.)

In general we think of all other living beings other than man, as indivisible from nature. They are a part of the system and cannot be conceived of as being against nature. It is only man that can. To say that man is part of nature too is a generalisation. Added to this is the point that man clearly does not really understand very much about nature, mainly because of his greed. As a result nature is exploited in a fashion that does not take care of the environment, especially among the so-called first world countries. The inhabitants of Asia have had fairly ecologically sound agricultural practices for well over 4,000 years. It is rather naïve to propose that only our modern standards have any scientific value, while denying this to those that have been practising scientifically sound methods for so long. The absence of a scientific doctrine for a particular method does not make it unscientific. And do we really believe that our standards will stand the test of time?

Since Galileo and Newton, our theories have undergone so many changes, that such a notion of lasting scientific values is at best an exercise in self-deception. We do not really know when agriculture began, and we assume from the ancient records that it is around the same time that man began to write. It is, therefore, perilous to assume that we can say anything definitive about the beginnings of agriculture, simply because we were not there to witness it.

The basic uncertainty is that we do not know what we mean by beginnings. Beginnings are always connected with ends, so that the state of fluctuation forms the stability of the system. The I Ching is based on the same principle; the changes are the only universal constant. Fluctuation implies relationship, because there is movement or flow between the living beings in an ecosystem. As man exploits nature he disturbs the flow by disharmoniously interfering with nature. Man is at war with nature but he can do much better if he treats her as a lover. In the not too distant past, a momentum took hold that was to lead western man more and more into the desire to control nature, rather than to assist her in submission. Like any other animal, man too can only continuously crop the surplus of plants for his food if ever he wants to survive. Harvesting the wild can be regarded as another form of natural death within the natural system. Because man has been endowed with intelligence, he can fool nature. By adapting natural principles like spacing and variety, man can create an environment which so resembles the natural state that pest and disease problems can be a thing of the past.

Meanwhile, in the prevalent system of agriculture, there exist alternative ways of getting rid of the pests and diseases that deserve the urgent attention of the public and a lift on the gag imposed on them becoming accepted practice. The NRA (Australian National Registration Authority) fees for registration of an agricultural pest, disease, or weed control product are, at $2,000 - a hindrance for small alternative businesses. The proposed increase to $20,000 will effectively push the small manufacturer of sustainable products out of the market. If this is the tactic the NRA employs, the prospects for the sustainability business look very bleak indeed.

Because knowledge like this is readily available to everyone, ICI, Ciba-Geigy, Rhone-Poulenc, and other chemical giants know this too. They usually debunk it as hogwash, the "return to the last century", or the dreaming of hippies. Sustainable agriculture does not represent a return to conservation-minded farming techniques without modern technologies. Sustainable systems use modern equipment, certified seed, soil and water, as well as livestock. Emphasis is placed on rotating crops, building up soil, diversifying crops and livestock and controlling pests naturally. Meanwhile, the pesticide manufacturers have seen that it works, and that the alternative bug sprays are too cheap to add to their own arsenal because there is no profit in them. Yet at the same time, by allowing the manufacturing by others, they would lose a big chunk of the market. Stringent fertiliser and pesticide acts make it harder for the alternative industry to have their products registered. Because the legislation clearly mentions minimum levels of NPK, any product that falls below the minimum levels is not allowed as fertiliser. Similarly, a bug spray based on garlic, which has proven to be reasonably effective, cannot, under present legislation, be registered as a pesticide. This reeks of a violation of the laws governing trusts and monopoly. Politically, little or nothing is done, although more and more evidence becomes available about the health aspects connected with pesticide and herbicide use. Which party will be able to sell the ideas of paying for the cost of diseases, caused by the use of excessive chemical poisons of Class 6 & 7?

The Chemical Method

From the brochure published by the Department of Agriculture, "Chemical control of insect pests in field crops and pasture" 1994, we can learn the following:

"The poison Schedule for each product is indicated in the table. Extremely toxic chemicals are labelled as 'dangerous poison' and belong to the class S7. The minimum protective clothing to be used when dealing with this class of chemicals is a suitable respirator and full protective clothing including a hood that covers the head."

Class S6, moderately toxic chemicals, is labelled 'poison'. A suitable respirator and protective clothing are required for spraying; goggles are also required for mixing the concentrate. For more detailed information on toxicity and safe handling, see Bulletin 4223, "Toxicity of pesticides" and Miscellaneous publication 8/88, "The toxicity of pesticides to wildlife". (Dept. of Agriculture WA.)

There is, on top of that, a 'withholding period' which indicates the time the crop has to be held by the farmer before he is allowed to sell it in the market. This is done to allow the sprays to be washed off by rain or to lose their toxicity over that period, as many modern pesticides have a short half-life. The products into which they are broken down are often equally toxic, but over a relatively short period only. All in all, in regards to the safety of modern pesticides, herbicides and fungicides it is not a rosy picture.

Anyone who wants to trial some product, even if it contains no toxins, has to obtain a license to do so from the NRA, with the exception of anything you try in your own backyard. Because of the links with the chemical companies, all alternatives to poisonous pesticides, insecticides & herbicides are treated with either suspicion or derision. This is governed by the fear of losing a market-share big enough to dent the profits. Yet one could argue that the organic or sustainable profits amount to little more than a drop in the ocean. However, the losses they have suffered already in Asia, to the tune of 13 million, may explain their increasing agitation.

Every day we can read in the papers how crops fail because of diseases and pests. The devastation by the fruit fly of the papaw crop is a stark example. The growers' answer is found in the advice from the pesticide manufacturer, which is to spray ever-deadlier poisons in ever-greater quantities.

At the same time parents get up in arms regularly over the spraying of playgrounds where toddlers – who are known to get into the dirt to the point of sticking it in their mouths – only a few hours later happily do just that. Considering the poisonous nature of the chemicals used, the parents' wrath is certainly justified.

In Europe, the use of sprays in parks is strictly regulated, although some countries have more stringent rules than others. The European consumer does no longer condone the massive use of sprays. In the Netherlands virtually every town has at least a health food store or supermarket, while in Amsterdam every suburb has at least a health food store. Among the growers of food crops, 12% have already made the switch to fully organic and sustainable methods while a further 40% are in the process of conversion. This means that over 50% of Dutch produce is grown without the use of chemical fertilisers, pesticides, herbicides and fungicides. Although the yields may be slightly smaller in the beginning, the money saved on chemicals more than compensates for the loss. Denmark is about to vote in a referendum to have a total ban on chemical controls of pests, diseases, and weeds, as well as chemical fertilisers.

In the US, the USDA estimates that between 60,000 to 100,000 farmers – about 3% of the nation's total – are practising non-conventional agriculture, most of which can be labelled sustainable. Among the consumers there is a growing cross-section which question the environmental, social, and economic impacts of conventional or chemical agriculture. As a consequence many farmers and other individuals are looking for alternative practices which could lead to increased sustainability.

Again in the US, this time in California, the consumers have mounted an attack on the manufacturers. This has resulted in the withdrawal of some 200 pesticide licenses. Although this is quite an achievement, much needs to be done to stop the use of these substances altogether. Any ideas that promote other ways of looking at the pesticide and herbicide problems will understandably be received with hostility by such firms as ICI, Ciba-Geigy, Rhone-Poulenc and others. Their answer will be that genetic engineering and biological control already help the farmer to get away from the use of highly toxic sprays. Although this looks at first sight to be a reasonable proposition, it is conveniently forgotten that these methods have still to prove their worth over a long period of time.

Genetic Engineering and Biological Control

At the moment, the push is for genetic engineering, as well as biological control. In the UK, as well as the Netherlands, firms have been established where natural predators are bred on a large scale, for a host of pests. This is, for Australian problems, of little significance, because of strict quarantine laws. The time needed to screen a predator for diseases would render them redundant for treatment of pests. The CSIRO has, moreover, its own breeding program. But if the experience with the cane toad is anything to go by, the introduction of a predator is fraught with its own difficulties. All too often the predator can become a pest in its own right, witness also the fox.

It may be appropriate to say something here about biological control methods.

1. Difficulties in rearing.
Some biological controls are difficult to rear. Fungi need specific moisture as well as a host. Predators need the same prey as they are supposed to control. Parasites do not survive very long or are cannibalistic.

2. Difficulties in keeping.
Some fungi do not keep very well. Predators need a host and a prey, while parasites need these facilities as well.

3. Effectiveness.
Fungi need moisture to be viable. Predators usually develop slower than pests. Parasites do not have these problems. All three are very species-specific and, as a consequence, they are not always effective.

4. Cost.
Many biological agents must be applied regularly from 1 to 4 weeks apart. They are expensive and sometimes not economically viable.

5. Resistance.
Most do not produce resistance, with the exception of the fungi.

"The dream of genetic engineering embodies the fallacy of a living system without time," as Gordon Harrison so aptly puts it. "In the short view stability in natural systems remains real and as valuable in maintaining the production of the earth, as instability is disastrous. The fact that one can see how it works may misleadingly suggest a machine that could be instantly reproduced."

The farmer, who tries to replace trees with corn and/or beans, quickly discovers that the abundant productivity of the forest cannot be simply re-channelled out of wood into crops. This leads to the drive to replace that abundance with 'Super' and NPK, which may give accelerated growth but, in reality, produce obese plants with little or no resistance. In turn these crops attract pests which are the predators of the plant world. The conventional answer to pests is the use of poisonous chemical sprays, which, when no longer effective, are at present to be replaced by genetic engineering. The ramifications and repercussions of that path are at the moment little, if at all understood. Fears that genetically implanted resistance to herbicides in food crops may cross over into the weeds that 'need to be killed', may not be without grounds. Given the results so far, it can be safely stated that the technique has not yet lived up to the promises made and has not delivered the goods.

The introduction of the soil bacterium Bacillus thuringiensis looked at first to be very promising. It appeared to kill serious pests like caterpillars, beetles and fly larvae, while being non-toxic to humans, spiders and other predators. By transferring the genes and encoding these in crop plants, it was assumed that the plants themselves would be the insecticides. Hence 'no-spray' cotton, potatoes or corn, cultivated in what was thought to be the Utopian farm.

At this moment it has to be admitted that what first looked so promising, is rapidly proving to be a lot less rosy. A handful of pests have already developed resistance against the 'pesticide plant', something the scientists had predicted would never happen. And according to the latest laboratory reports, many other pests like the Colorado beetle and some species of budworm, have the potential to become resistant in the near future. The worry is really that by putting toxic genes into crops, the evolution of 'superbugs', resistant to an array of transgenic toxins, might be encouraged much sooner than previously thought.

The reaction is more of the same; to outwit the evolution and forestalling resistance. What strikes one as dimwitted is the fact that what has already proven not to work is now pursued with even more vigour. It is an observable fact that in the last 50 years developments in pest control have followed the same patterns, governed by the assumption that resistance could be overcome by either more or stronger versions of the same substances. The trend has now shifted to genetic engineering backed by the same fallacious philosophy. Although bacterial toxins are a lot more selective in what they kill, the burgeoning business they have generated is exactly what fans the worry about resistance. In the 1980s their sales have increased more than fourfold, to the tune of over US $100 million. Although farmers have been abundantly spraying Bt, as it is called, for over 20 years, without there ever being any evidence of resistant insects, that picture is fast being demolished. Some scientists have always been skeptics. Whenever there is a new insecticide, people think of reasons why it is impossible for insects to become resistant to it. Others just assume they are going to become resistant, which is a safer viewpoint.

As early as 1985, the first resistant moths taken from grain storage bins in the Midwestern US were identified. Then in 1990, scientists came across another moth, the diamondback, on Hawaiian cabbage and watercress. Consequently, resistant diamondbacks have been found as far afield as Florida, New York State, Japan and mainland Asia. Roughly a dozen breeding experiments have only confirmed that a wide range of insects has the capacity to develop resistance. On top of that, the toxins lose their potency in a couple of days after spraying, because of sunlight which breaks them down rapidly. Thus the protection they provide is only very temporary.

Transgenic cotton and potatoes are already a fact and so are tomatoes, while maize and soybeans should follow shortly. While it looks as though this development might be sensible to get rid of pests, the risk of resistant survivors passing on their resistance to their progeny increases with every generation. If it were not for transgenic plants there would not be such an urgent need to deal with the resistance problem. Other critics accuse Monsanto, the producer of Bt, of dragging its feet. It is the old style of working – it is studied to death. By the time resistance appears it is too late. Scientists have to pay attention to clues that it is coming, or the battle is lost. It is scientific suicide to sit back and say, let's wait and see what is going on. At the same time, because of the complexities of the subject, scientists know little about which of their tactics might work. Scientists can model and discuss or try to run lab experiments, but it appears that they all agree that this is insufficient to come up with an answer that will allay the fears of the farmers.

Modern Farming Methods

Meanwhile, in Australia the farmers are still locked in the position of having to use chemical sprays, with the exception of the cotton growers. Some biological pest and weed control is being experimented with by the CSIRO. Too many farmers have the sword of bankruptcy hanging over their heads. The government has to give heavy subsidies to farmers. The chemical companies have the last laugh, as they are pocketing the money spent on their not so effective 'control'.

In Australia, farming is threatening to destroy the topsoil and the native flora and fauna over vast areas. Topsoil is generally very thin at about 1 centimetre and, therefore, is prone to wash away quite quickly. Together with the use of fertiliser and bare soil cultivation, the problem is compounded as the amount of organic matter in the soil is depleted to zero. The biggest problem is that the Australian landscape is not fit for European style agriculture. Land clearing to the tune of two football pitches per minute, or 500,000 ha per year, belongs to the worst record in the world. In 1990 alone, 650,000 ha were cleared which amounts to more than half the area cleared in the Amazon basin. In the past 50 years, as much land has been cleared as in the 150 years since settlement. In 1995 permits were granted to clear more than a million ha in Queensland alone, among which are 685,000 ha of virgin bush.

Land clearance has been very costly in terms of environmental damage. Rainfall has been reduced by 14%, adding to the desertification of Australia at a rate the country cannot really afford. Bio-diversity is another area that suffers greatly from European farming methods. Meanwhile the farmers consider it illogical to blame them. With the government giving tax incentives for clearing native bushland, their reaction is understandable. If, instead, the farmers would receive tax breaks to manage the land sustainably, they would do so, according to Robert Hadler of the National Farmers Federation. It is significant that 20% of the farmers grow enough food to sustain the whole population of Australia. The other 80% are subject to the international market forces, where the prices are set by the same companies that sell the seed of the hybrids which the farmers grow, making for a vice like grip they find themselves in.

About 30% of the landholders are members of Landcare, a network of more than 2,000 regional conservation groups. Yet the use of alternatives to fertilisers and pesticides is severely hampered by the NRA, the Fertiliser Act, as well as the Agricultural Chemicals Act. The first is manned by people with interests in the fertiliser and chemical control industry, while the latter two forbid the use of alternatives.

What has happened so far is that farmers have been hitting pests as hard as possible, with high doses of pesticides. The reasoning behind it is that if they are hit hard enough, those that have a little resistance will also be killed. In this way they try to stop the passing on of resistance to the next generation. The problem with this is that it has to be done perfectly, which is virtually impossible in the field as the conditions in nature are <u>always</u> less than perfect. If there are any survivors from such high dose strategy they are going to be highly resistant. To date, no pesticide has ever been able to wipe out every member of an insect population. Experience has shown that it is the quickest way to create resistant pests. Tobacco budworm has already proven to be resistant to several species of Bt, even when sprayed simultaneously. The latest strategy involves Integrated Pest Management, or IPM, where sparingly used sprays, crop rotation, natural enemies and altered planting dates, to miss pest breeding cycles, are used to avoid the development of pest resistance. Although this is a much more sensible approach, it still misses the essential point.

A Real Alternative

If the whole issue is viewed from the idea that the pest is the problem, the wild goose chase will go on *ad infinitum*. There will be no solutions, only more lost battles, till the war with pests is lost and the world populations succumb to famine. What has been lacking so far is the notion that the plant is having the problem. Although genetic engineering seems to tackle that, it is still only done to get at the pest indirectly.

The conclusion to be drawn from this is that the approach to pest management has to move in a new direction. Both farmers and consumers want food that has been grown under optimum circumstances and conditions. This does not always mean the biggest grains, fruits and vegetables without any blemishes. Optimum growth is what occurs in perfectly natural circumstances. It is possible only in a subtly and organically attuned environment. Plants will always attract pests and diseases. It is time we learn to accept that our unrealistic expectations in this regard have to be abandoned. Still, we have to address the problems of pests and diseases. It is imperative to look at what is really happening.

To understand the incidence of disease and the susceptibility to pests requires the abandonment of the idea of control per se, as a goal in itself. It requires a new paradigm that takes into account the facts rather than conjecture, speculation and theory. Far from being rational, the efforts have always focused on the pest or disease as the problem. *In reality it is the plant that suffers from them, therefore it is the plant that needs treatment*. This is the only rational approach. The causes have to be removed, which will be outlined below under the heading 'soil structure and plant physiology'. If this is not possible, as is the case with the massive crops the modern farmer needs to grow if his business is to be viable, then the homoeopathic approach allows him at least to be free of toxic sprays. The very small doses make it safe, environmentally friendly, non-toxic, frugal with resources and extremely cheap, if only because one application is generally sufficient. Because it treats the plant, it enhances its immune system, which trait could very well be passed on to the next generation without the need for genetic engineering. Also, the pests do not develop resistance since they are no longer the targets. The benefits to both the primary producer and the consumer are self-evident.

When a pest is sprayed, all that is achieved is thinning the local pest population. This invites other members of the same species to fill the gap, so little more than a delay in pest attack is achieved. Homoeopathic remedies treat the plant, not the pest or disease. This results in stronger, healthier plants, unacceptable to pests and not prone to disease attack.

Inter-cropping with companion plants deserves much more attention than it gets. Yet very few farmers use the companion plant method, as harvesting machinery is not equipped for dual tasks. For monoculture farming the homoeopathic approach is the best possible answer.

Homoeopathic medicine applies remedies in very small doses – much smaller than conventional and even biodynamic methods – so no harmful residues are built up within the environment. Even highly toxic substances such as arsenic, become virtually harmless in highly diluted form, but remain effective in plants that suffer from pest- or disease-attack. Plants only absorb micro-doses of any substance, hence a homoeopathic remedy is particularly adapted for the treatment of plants. Both as a spray and in the trickle system, a remedy is absorbed in the shortest possible time. Both the leaves and the roots absorb a remedy well.

Homoeopathic medicine is readily available worldwide. It has no limitations on shelf life. Its effectiveness is unparalleled, as generally one dose is sufficient to give protection to the plant during its entire lifecycle, at least in annuals and biennials. Resistance is never a problem, because it aims at the plant rather than the disease or pest. The price is negligible compared to chemical treatment or even biological control.

An Example

In addition to 6 biological controls, such as predators, chrysanthemum growers use 2 sprays of Bt. and 4 to 6 pesticides. These have to be sprayed regularly from 1 to 4 weeks apart. If they were to use homoeopathic remedies, they need no more than 4 remedies maximum, which need to be sprayed only once and only if a pest attack is already happening. *If he uses a remedy made from the companion plant, he needs only 1 remedy for all the problems met with in his crop and that only in a single dose.* The difference is obvious. Instead of using sprays between 12 to 16 times, this is reduced to a maximum of 4 and a minimum of 1. This is a reduction of at least 70% and at best 98% in the work involved, while the cost goes down more considerably even when they need 4 remedies. The savings are about 90%. The only drawback lays in the antidotal relationship between the remedies used which, therefore, may need repetition and will increase his costs by a small margin.

To understand what this entails in regards to the remedies we have to look at their sources and the function they have in plant-life in general. Also we have to look at the immediate environment in which the plant grows. Thus above ground, we have first of all the plants themselves, both the crop and the "weeds". A further component is the weather and the climate; the first the local situation from day to day, the second the weather pattern over a long period. Then the situation on the ground demands our attention; the soil-type, its structure, the humus content, the pH, and the presence of weeds. The type of cultivation, i.e. bare soil, organic, permaculture, biodynamic, biological or conventional, plays an equally important role. In bare soil cultivation the fungi, bacteria and viruses which are, in reality, soil borne and provide the function of decomposers in a natural setting, are forced to attack living plants to guarantee their survival.

Under the surface of the soil, microbial life is necessary for the processing of the organic nutrients so they become available to plants. In conventional agriculture the nutrients are applied in soluble inorganic form which promotes leaching and makes it hard to maintain optimum nutrient levels throughout the life of the plant.

The remedies come from three different sources and their action is dependent on the source. The tissue salts are, from their action, related to diseases, as is evident from the symptoms produced. The particular nutrient excesses and deficiencies and the relationships between the different nutrients, such as the inimical, the complementary, the antidote and comparisons are described in some detail.

We can, therefore, conclude that for instance potassium, which fixes phosphorus, is in that case the antidote to it, because it stops the action of phosphorus. At the same time it can be argued that they are inimical, because potassium obviously acts here as an inimical substance.

In regards to the tissue salts it is noteworthy that the so called macro-nutrients appear to have been given the most attention and have been presented as the most important mainly because they are present in the greatest quantity. If we look however at the micro-nutrients, we see that an imbalance has much more devastating effects on a plant than an imbalance of the NPK group. Just like a human being can have a deficiency in food and survive very well, a plant can handle an imbalance of the plant foods N, P, or K, much better than an imbalance of, for example, boron which immediately produce more dangerous symptoms. Therefore, I propose that the micro-nutrients are regarded as essential remedies, while the members of the macro-nutrient group are given second rank in this materia medica.

The remedies derived from plants are more suited to pests, although some of them, especially the companion plants, are also effective against diseases, particularly on their companion. There they function like a constitutional remedy, as all symptoms that the companion produces are covered by the protective plant. An example is *Ocymum*, which is the companion to tomato, and which will protect the tomato against all pests and diseases pertaining to it.

The remedies made from the invertebrates such as insects and gastropoda are either very specific, or generic. *Helix* is specific against snails and slugs, while *Bombyx* is generic against caterpillars. Sometimes these remedies can act also against diseases, but only if the symptoms resemble the damage done by the pest from which they are made.

Soil, weather, crop and biome are the four legs of the stool of diagnosis, which can be extended with laboratory reports and microscopic evidence.

Soil Structure and Plant Physiology

True science requires that the subject under investigation is studied in its totality. All attempts at isolation and reduction of the related parts, renders the scientific endeavour to a meaningless mumbo-jumbo of unrelated events. The homoeopathic approach to the problems met with in growing plants, whether for food or as an exercise in recreation, is scientific in the true sense of the word. It studies pests, diseases, and soil problems as symptoms of a totality within the environment. The totality includes the medium in which the plant grows, the climate and weather patterns, the availability of water, nutrients and the occurrence of other organisms in that whole environment which is the local ecosystem.

The Soil

Looking at a vertical section of soil, the first thing that demands the attention is the variation of colour and a certain amount of dead organic matter, a host of living entities, structure and porosity as well as the extent of weathering and erosion. These elements form distinct layers which are known as horizons. Three of these are usually taken into account.

Topsoil

This is the upper region where the greatest biological, physical, and chemical activity takes place. The major portion of living entities, organic matter, and chemical reaction are found here. A host of insects, earthworms, protists, nematodes and decomposer organisms all contribute to the decomposition of leaves, twigs, bark and wood.

Second Horizon.

This is the layer where nutrients and small particles of organic matter are deposited. This process uses percolation, or moving down through the soil. It is self evident that much less organic matter is available, while erosion is reduced to a minimum.

Elimination

The lowest horizon is where excess elements are leached out. It consists of larger particles of rock of any one kind, sand, lime or basalt, to name but a few, gravel and other debris. For the purpose of this book only the two top layers are of significance.

Dependent on the amount of organic matter, a soil is either a sponge or it is not. From an ecological point of view, bare soil cultivation, with little or no organic content, adds to global warming because of its low water retention properties. A soil that acts as a sponge cools down the air directly above it, thus helping plants to cope better with heat, reducing evaporation from both the soil and the plant. Reflection is reduced to the minimum possible if sufficient organic matter is suspended in the soil, while the lack of it increases reflection of heat. Also dependent on the content of organic matter is the determination about the quality of the soil - whether it is active or passive. Modern agricultural practises have produced vast tracts of passive soils, because nutrients have been given priority in the growth of plants. Soil is however much more than a medium in which to suspend nutrients.

Dead soils - the ultimate in passivity - have no organic content. This can support little if any microbial life which, for want of its proper food source, will attack living plants, creating a host of plant diseases, while the insects are more or less forced into a similar pattern of survival. To reverse this position requires a drastic turn of events if the agricultural endeavour is to produce healthy crops and turn it into a viable economic and ecological enterprise.

Soil is very dependent on light and air, however strange this may appear. Air and light are usually associated with above ground phenomena. Yet without light and air, even in the soil, essential elements to life are absent which plants require for their immune systems. Science knows much more about the part of plants which grows above ground than about the roots, although this picture is changing fast. The processes in the roots are fairly well known, but little is known about the interaction of soil and root. The emphasis is placed on the nutrients, while the pH - the acidity or alkalinity of the soil - is studied only in the context of the nutrient levels. Structure, biological activity and organic content are studied only in relation to these same levels, while the knowledge thus gathered is used only to 'improve' the manufacture, synthetic or otherwise, of the nutrients.

The homoeopathic approach is systemic - it does not compartmentalise the soil into plants and nutrients, nor does it limit itself to organic content and biomass. Although they are essential building blocks forming a healthy soil, other non visible elements, perceivable only by their results, are included as well.

Organic Matter

This consists of plant debris, dead animals, insects, and other biological entities. This forms the food of a host of other insects such as ants, slaters, snails and slugs, many fungi, moulds and mildews, bacteria and viruses. Collectively, these organisms are called decomposers - they break down organic matter into smaller particles and compounds, which in turn are processed into the various nutrients. They are always in relation to and in connection with the organisms which produce them. These organisms release these nutrients in a steady stream to feed the plants. Fine particles of organic matter cling to the roots and any plant is a decomposer in its own right. The roots, through the process of growth, bring light and air into the soil, together with the rest of the biomass. Micro-organisms are of two types; aerobic and anaerobic, the former needs air to function properly, while the latter needs carbon-dioxide for the same purpose.

Insects

Many of the 'pests', identified because of their habit to feed on our food crops, are actually supposed to feed on organic debris, just as that is the function of fungi, bacteria and viruses. In the absence of dead organic matter these organisms are forced to feed on living plants in order to correct the imbalance created by bare soil cultivation. In nature, the sum total of events is designed to maintain balance. Balance means even spacing, because it will prevent the crowding of one particular species. Monocultures are designed to outdo natural arrangements. Space in nature tends to be occupied by as great a variety as the natural habitat allows. Through this mechanism nature limits disease and the consequent elimination of any one species of plant, insect or animal. Too many plants or animals of the same species occupying too small a space triggers the mechanism that prevents breeding and makes up for excess through more rapid death, by means of pests and diseases.

All stable natural systems have those switches, but not all populations do. In Australia we see this in the rapid explosion of the rabbit populations. In agriculture, species like the locust, the aphid or the Colorado beetle, rodents like rats and mice, display the phenomenon, that, when provided with sufficient food, will rapidly produce enormously more young than the available food supply. A farmer sowing a crop of their favourite food supply, creates a situation where there is a massive reduction in the infant mortality rate of the pest.

Fluctuation implies relationship, because there is a flow between the living beings in an ecosystem. As man exploits nature he disturbs the flow, when his dealings are disharmonious. Thus man is at war with nature, while he could do much better if he sees her as a lover. Harvesting from nature can be seen as another form of natural death within an ecosystem, provided the spacing between plants is kept as natural as possible. In this way nature can be fooled into believing that harvesting is an absolutely natural occurrence, similar to grazing and foraging animals. To this end it is imperative that the immediate surroundings of food crops are as natural as possible.

Deposition

In the soil above this horizon the nutrients are deposited. In general ten of the elements are believed to be nutrients. About a hundred years ago, these ten elements - carbon, hydrogen, nitrogen, oxygen, potassium, calcium, magnesium, phosphorus, sulphur and iron - were designated as essential elements for plant growth. In the early 1900s manganese was added. The importance of silica has only recently, around 1985, received the full attention it deserves. At present we know that copper, boron and molybdenum play an important role as well, while for some plants cobalt and aluminium are necessary. In speaking of inorganic nutrients, it follows that there must be organic forms as well. Little is said about them in the textbooks, maybe due to the fact that inorganic chemistry is not interested in the investigation of the organic content of the elements.

Although chemical analysis is useful to determine the relative amounts of nutrients in certain stages of growth of the healthy plant in natural surroundings, it is by no means an exclusive yardstick, as different plants have different requirements in different ecosystems. Deficiencies will create havoc in equal manner as excesses. The homoeopathic approach requires that which is natural to a particular ecosystem.

In some, the soil may be dead as in the desert, or rich as in the rainforest. Soils are as individual as the plants that prefer a particular type. Thus the soil type is the first point of investigation, together with its structure and the amount of biomass. In the case of dead soils, much can be done to revive it by the selection of the appropriate remedy.

Nutrients

Most nutrients are essential for certain functions of plant life, be it photosynthesis, growth or metabolism. Some plants are characterised by unusual higher or lower concentrations of (a) particular nutrient(s). It is therefore self evident that plants have different requirements amongst each other, even if grown in the same medium. Because of the complexity of the bio-mass it may appear that, for instance, alfalfa benefits from a nitrogen boost, as it is a nitrogen fixing plant. However, alfalfa can only take up the nitrogen provided by soil-bacteria, which would suffer a redundancy with a nitrogen boost, leaving the plant nitrogen-deficient. Other plants, called C4 plants, require sodium instead of potassium, or at least to a greater extent. Atriplex also known as saltbush, is one of several halophytes which requires salt to grow properly. Salt is pumped from the leaf tissue through the stalk into large expanding bladder cells. Soybeans, when deprived of nickel, will develop toxic levels of urea, resulting in necrosis in the leaf tips, and reduce growth.

Inorganic ions affect osmosis and thus help water balance. (See *Natrum mur.* and others like *Sulphur* and the *Kali* preps.) Because several inorganic ions can serve this purpose, independent from each other, in many different plants, it is understood to be non-specific. On the other hand, an inorganic element may function as part of an essential biological molecule and as such its necessity is highly specific. As an example, magnesium presence in the chlorophyll molecule is highly essential to and in photosynthesis. Magnesium is strongly attracted to light and helps oxidation in the form of the oxide, thus enhancing oxygen production and release.

Some elements are essential to the structure of cell-membranes, while others control the function of these membranes, such as permeability. The enzyme systems in a plant require specific elements to be present, while others again provide the ionic tension required for certain biological reactions. Deficiencies affect a wide variety of structures and functions as do excesses. This is because they fill such basic needs and processes essential to healthy growth and strong immune systems in the plant body.

One of the key roles elements play, is in the participation as catalysts in enzymatic processes. They can be an essential part in the enzyme structure. They can also function as activators and regulators of enzymes. Potassium, for instance, is thought to be involved in some 50 to 60 enzymes and is believed to regulate the production of some proteins. As biologists look at the single elements, the interactions between different elements, such as the compounds, like nitrate of potassium or the phosphate of sodium are little understood. In the homoeopathic scenario, these differences in

(continued on page 36)

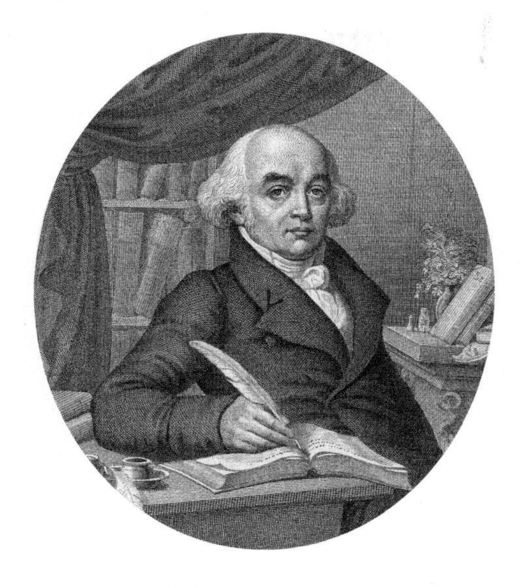

Homoeopathy has been used to treat humans since Hahnemann began his work in the 1800s.

There was already interest in using homoeopathy on the land in the 19th century, but nothing even remotely similar attained momentum until Dr. Rudolf Steiner gave his 'biodynamic' agricultural course in 1924.

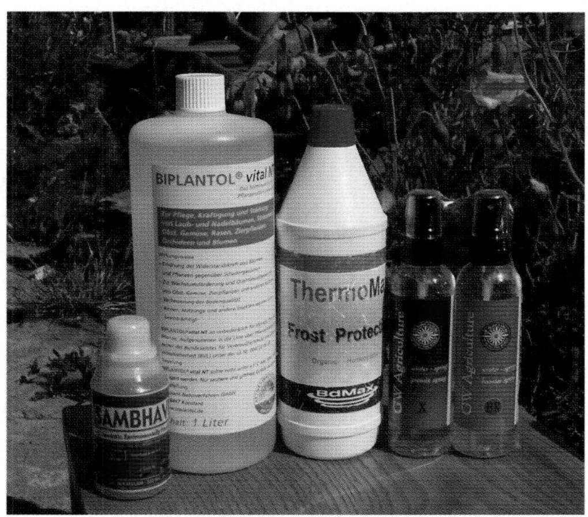

Now several homoeopathically prepared products are available for gardeners and farmers. Some are inspired by biodynamic agriculture, others by the classical homoeopathic tradition that has developed from the initiative of Hahnemann.

With so many remedies, plants, diseases, soils and climates, there is work to do to reveal the potential of using homoeopathy on the land.

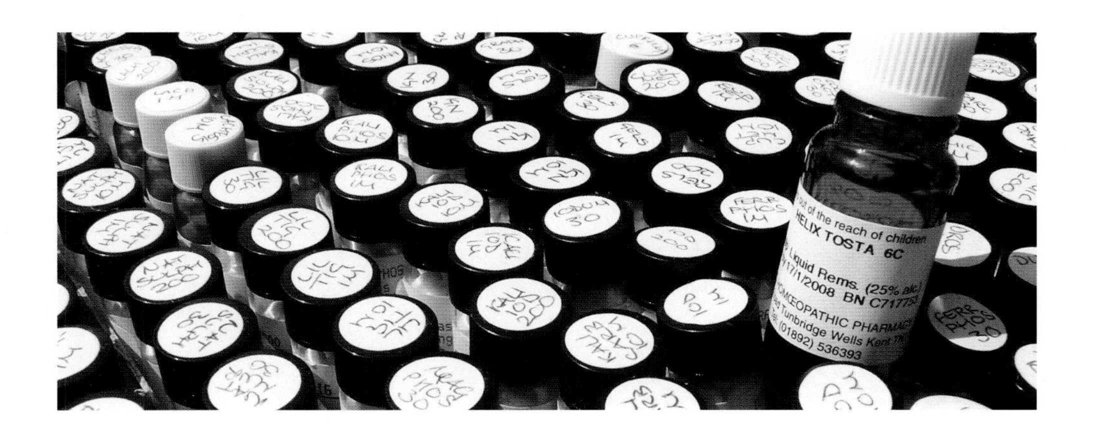

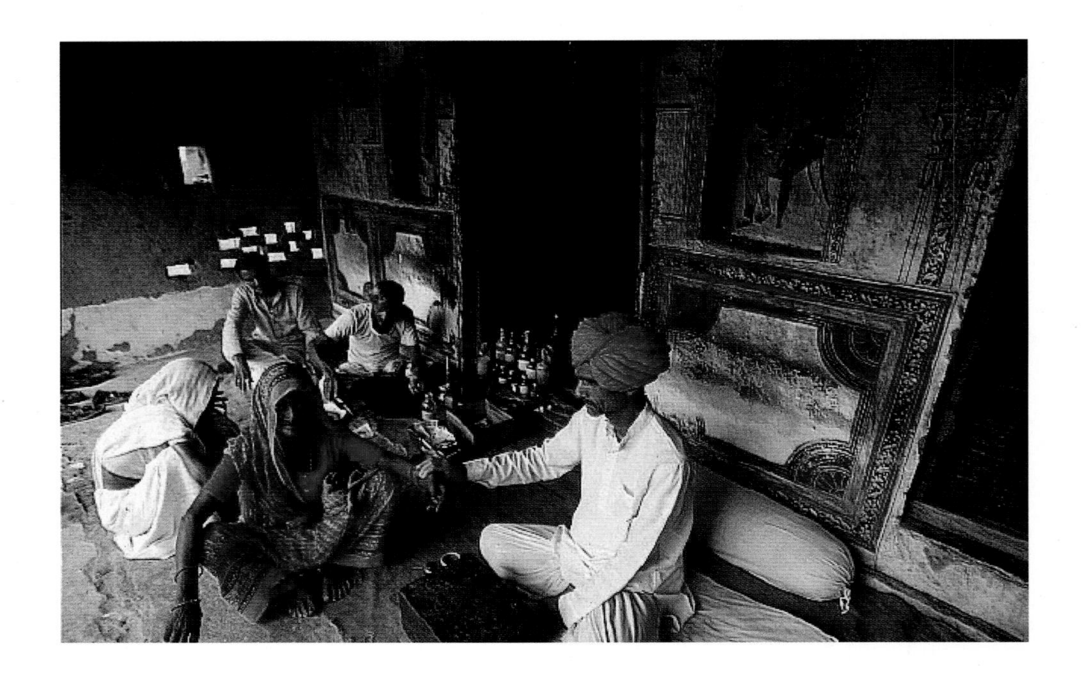

Homoeopathy for humans and animals is used across the world. Preparation of remedies can be as highly controlled as for any modern drug, but most remedies can be made in a verandah surgery or clean kitchen.

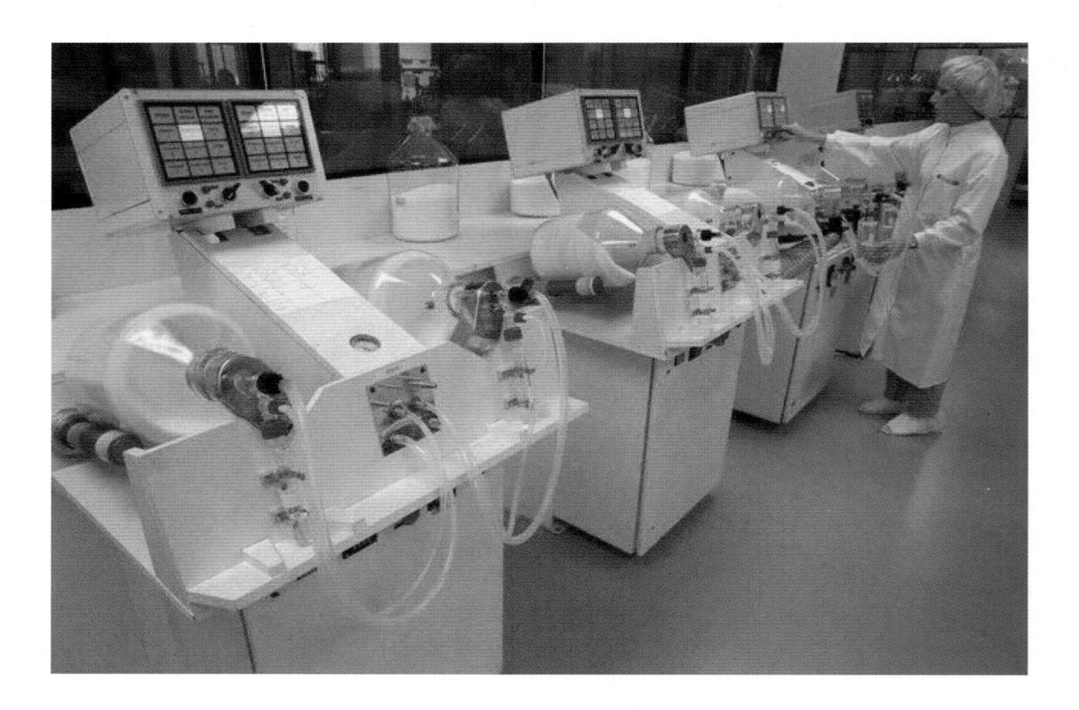

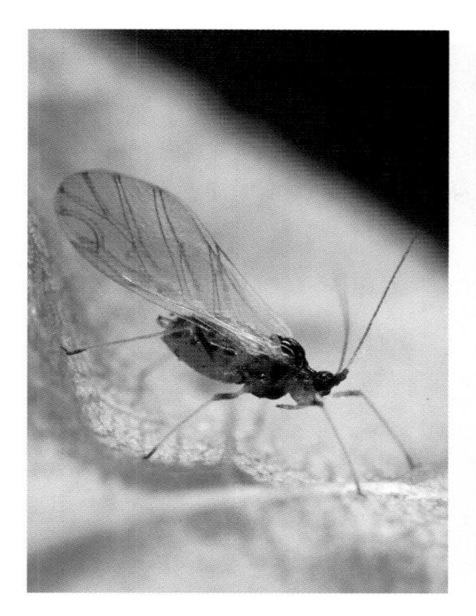

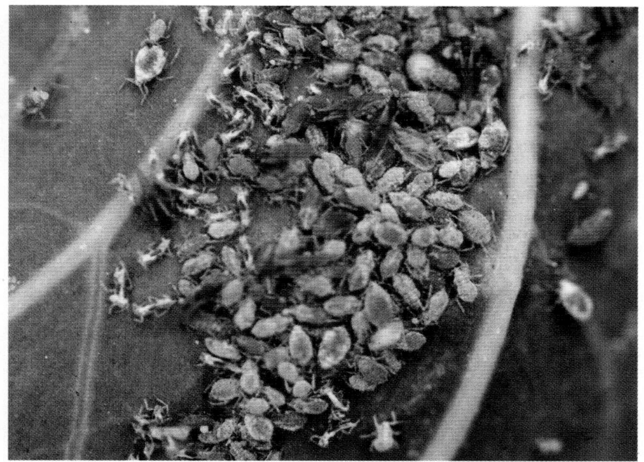

Homoeopathy does not consider the pest to be the root of the problem. The problem is that some plants are susceptible to the ubiquitous pests. The aphids seen here might leave one plant unscathed but devour its neighbour. Therefore, stricken plants need to be strengthened by good husbandry and by non-toxic remedies. In this light the pest is primarily an indicator of the state of health of the plant, and its proliferation is just one symptom to be taken into account with all the others that can be gleaned by careful observation. Several remedies have been shown to have some efficacy in turning vulnerable plants into resistant plants. It is interesting to note that the remedy made from the aphid-eating ladybird - *Coccinella Septempunctata* - is one of them. Is this a principle - homoeopathic integrated pest management (hIPM!) - that might be extended to plants susceptible to other pests?

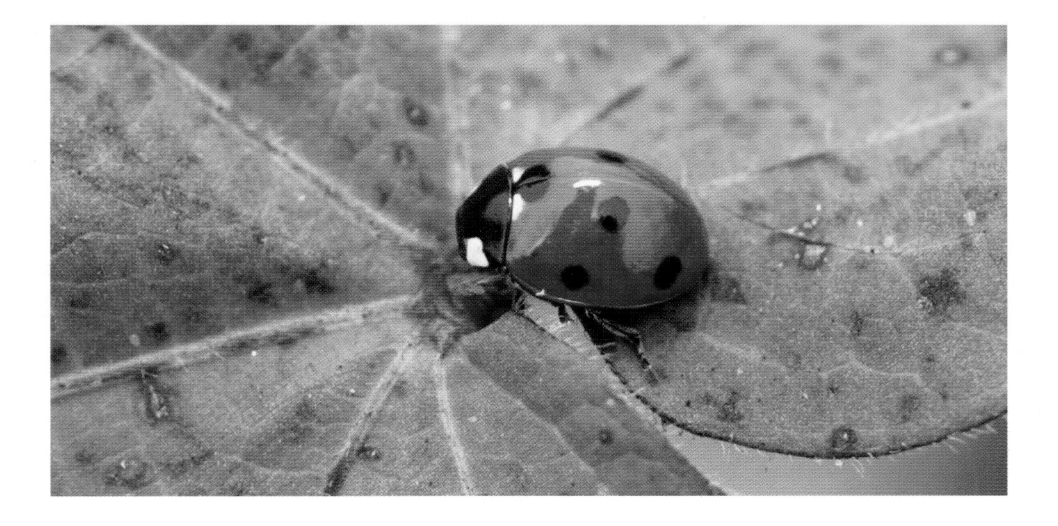

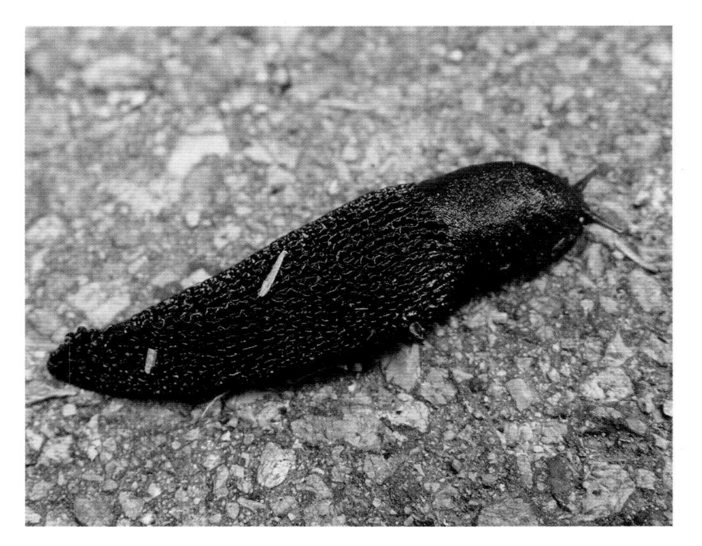

Gardeners always ask, 'What about slugs?' Look at the materia medica entry, on page 91, for *Helix Tosta* made from the common snail, and page 99 for *Kali permanganum.*

Some pests, when potentised, become the remedy to strengthen plants against themselves. *Helix Tosta* is also effective against snails, *Bombyx* against other caterpillars, and *Porcellio* against slaters. But aphids were not a particularly effective remedy against themselves. This 'isopathy' is used for humans, and even more so in veterinary homoeopathy. The extent of its role in farming and gardening remains to be discovered.

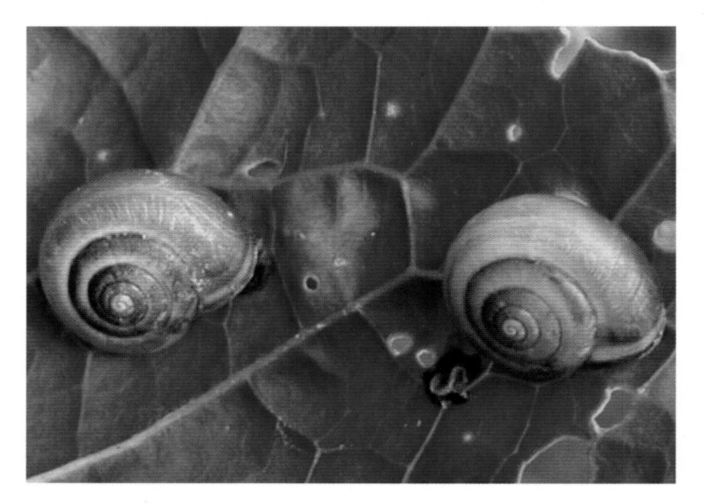

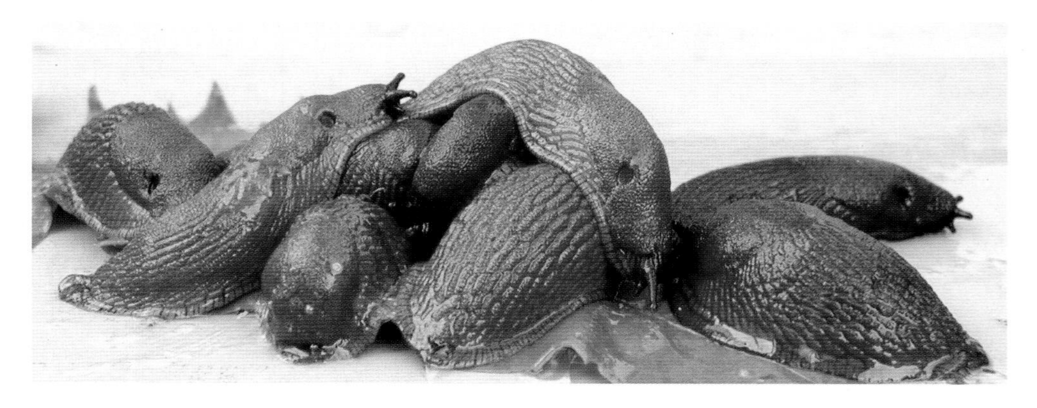

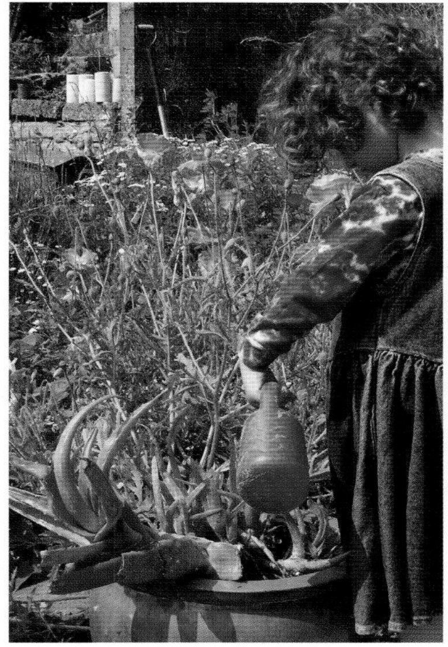

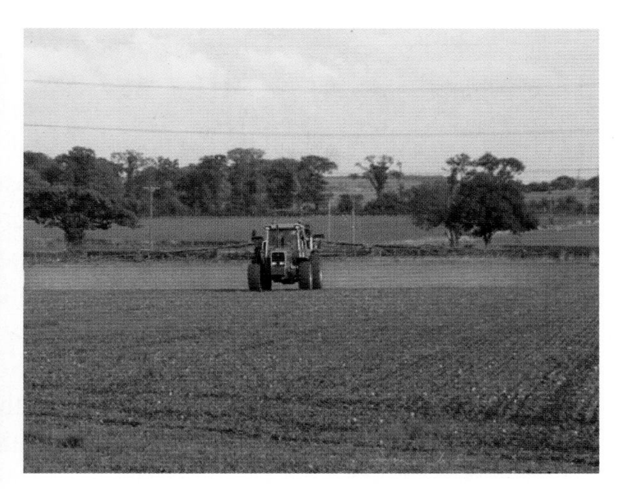

The remedies are simple to apply and safe enough to be handled by anyone. Remedies can be administered by hand, added to the irrigation water or applied through small or large sprayers. The machine below is using electrostatic attraction to make the droplets adhere to the tree and avoid drift in built up areas. (In this case the remedies are potentised biodynamic preparations used to boost the struggling horse chestnut trees in the Hague.)

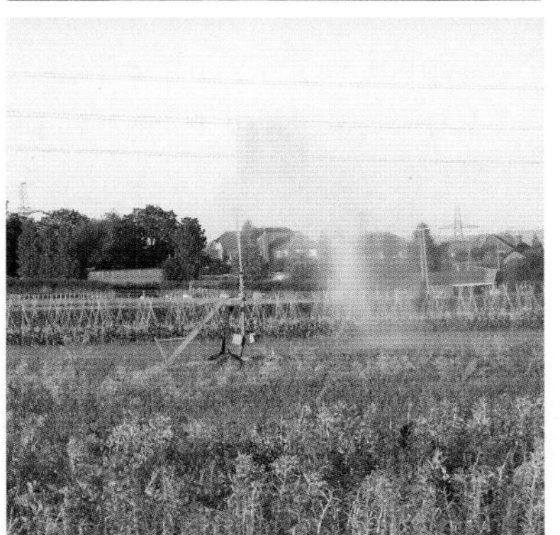

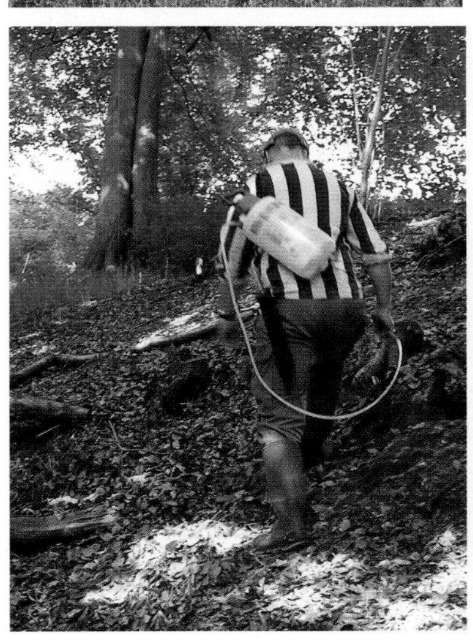

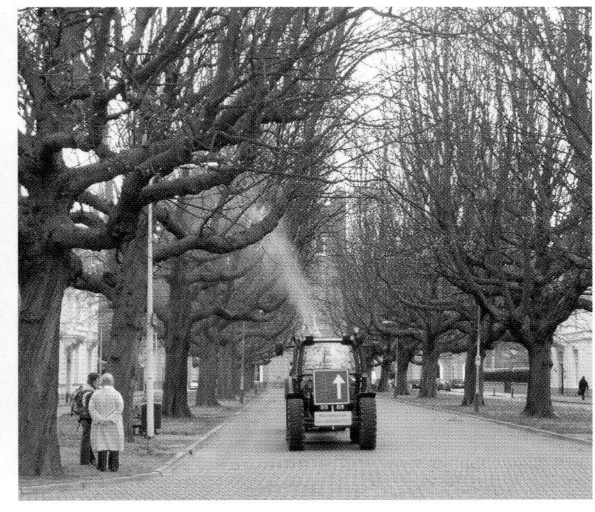

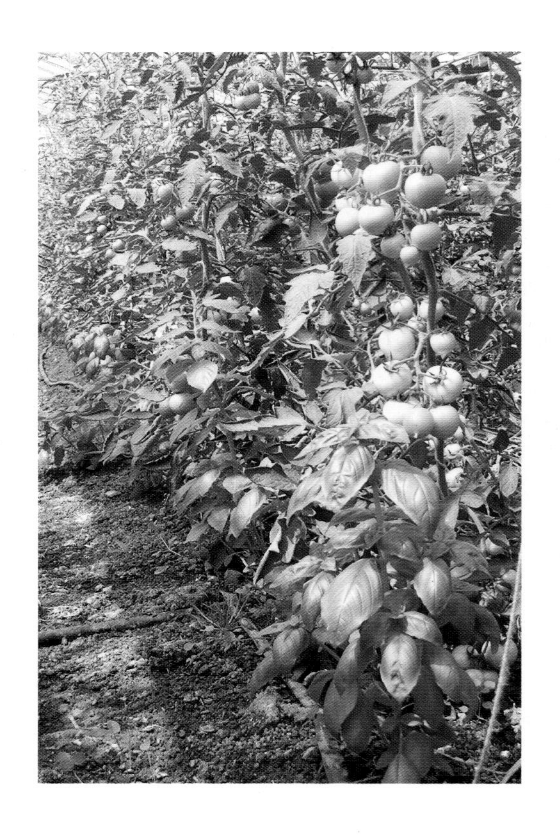

Homoeopathic medicine has developed as an empirical discipline working from tests ('provings') and collated experiences of successes and failures. If basic principles could be teased out from the experience with plants then one could select likely remedies for new situations with greater certainty. One of the ways considered is that of using potentised 'companion plants'. Here tomatoes are shown growing with basil to their mutual benefit. The homoeopathic version of the basil - *Ocymum Basilicum* - benefits tomatoes in many ways! It suggests itself as a kind of 'constitutional remedy' of the tomato plant.

Until such time as principles are identified with confidence, I will continue to experiment with nosodes, potentised predators (for example *Aranea Diadema* to the right) and companion plants, or use what anthropomorphic hints strike me. (The decision which started my experimentation - to try Belladonna on a thirsty cordon of apples affected by a virulent red rust - was made by analogy with humans.) But whatever inspiration or principle is used, one must practice close observation and experimental rigor to judge the successes and failures in any trials and experiments.

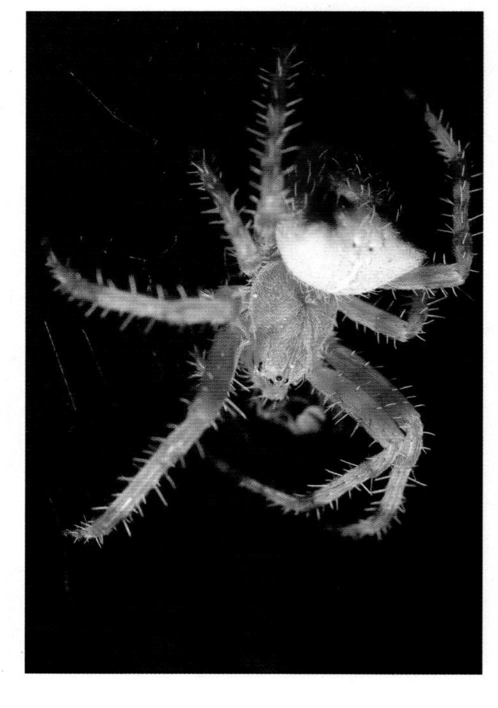

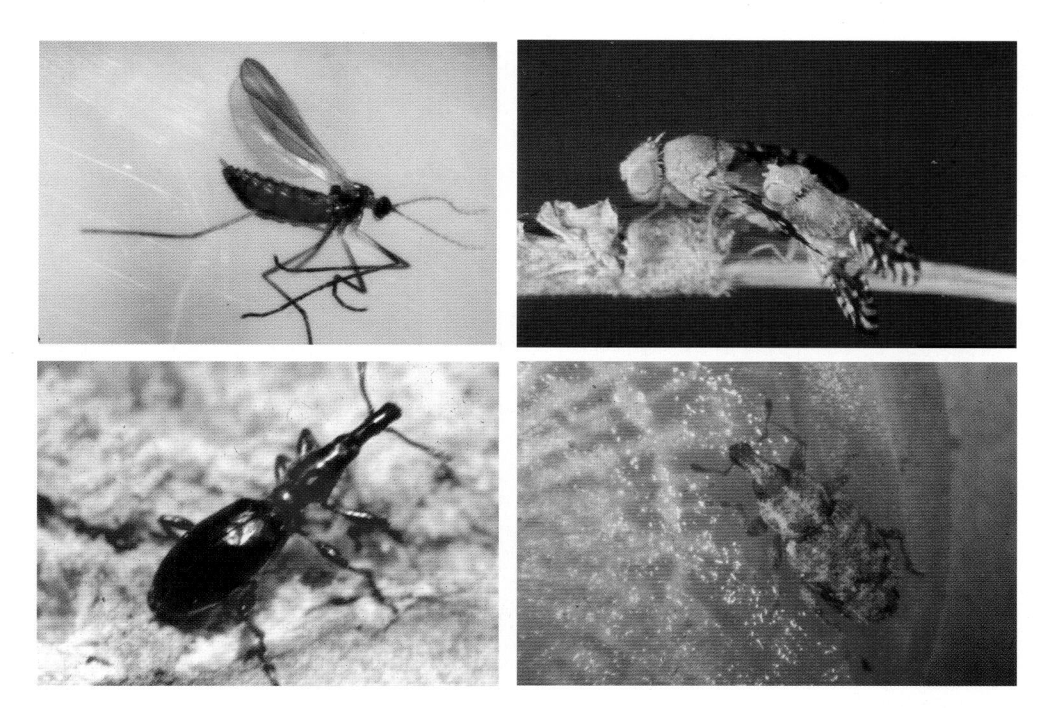

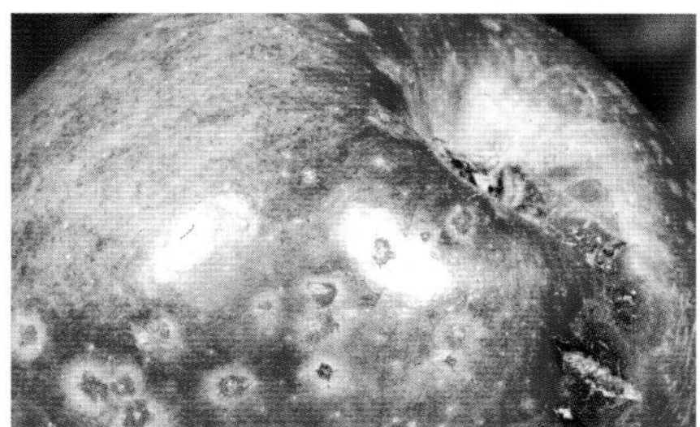

Observations which commonly occur together have already been identified. We know them as named diseases and pests. The materia medica and repertory make use of these, but also of individual aspects revealed directly to the unscholared eye, nose, tongue and finger.

The apple on the right is officially suffering from 'scab', the bean with 'anthracnose'. But we can also try and describe how that scab and anthracnose are manifesting using primary descriptive terms. Such 'unprejudiced observation' discourages lazy and inappropriate description, and keeps the discipline open to the non-academic.

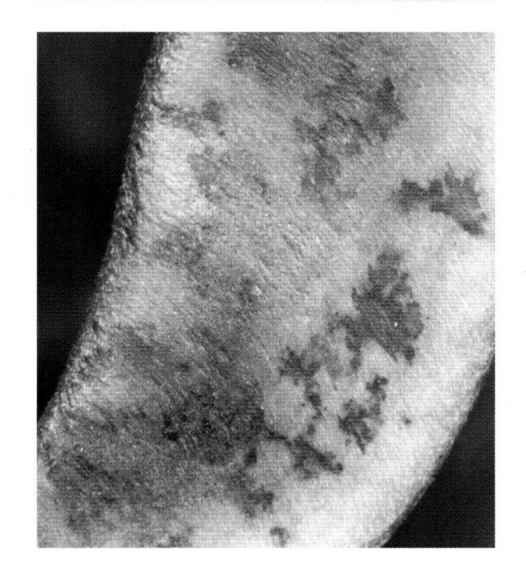

Although a diagnosis such as 'nematode' is a good start to selecting the right remedy, (our fledgling repertory suggests the following: **Calend**., Calc.fl., Calc.p., *Carbo v.,* Nast., Sul., **Tanac., Teuc.** Val. Zinc m.) all the images below show nematodes and their damage. One has to discriminate within those listed in the repertory by reading their entries in the materia medica.

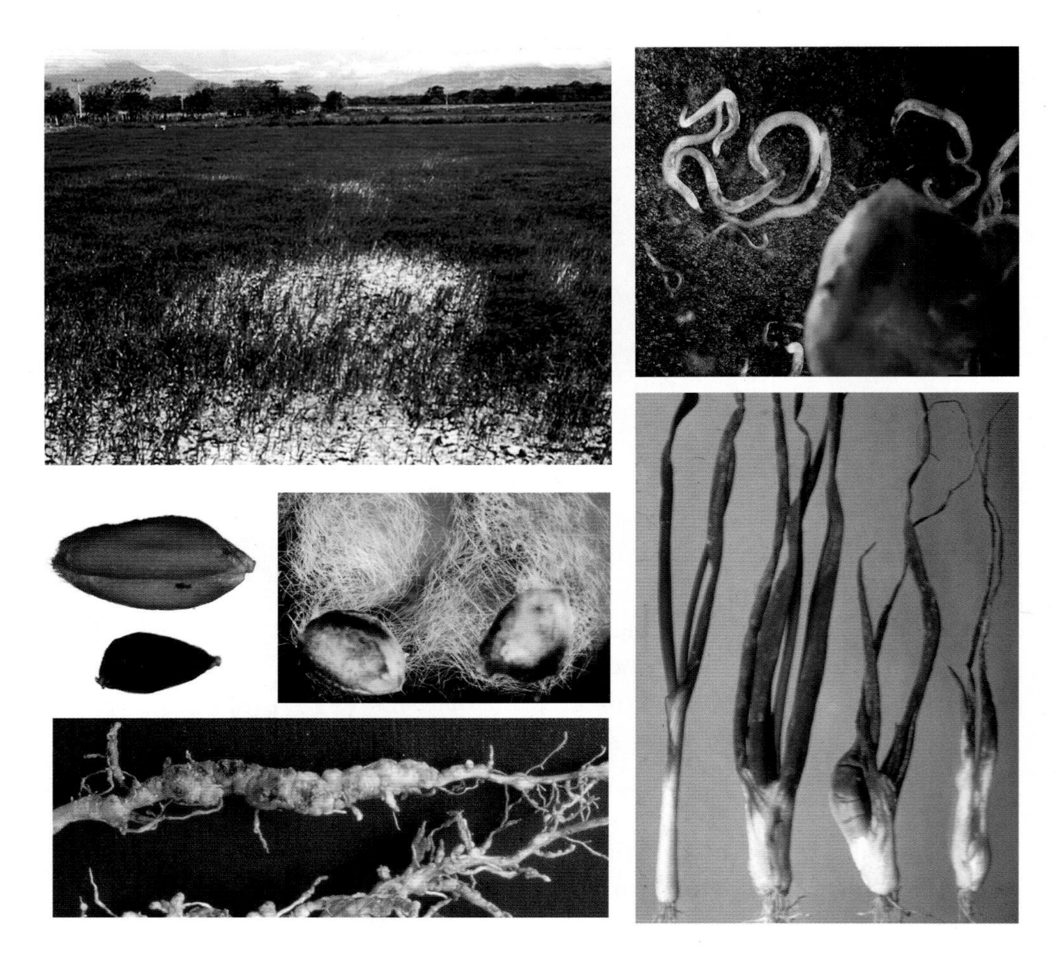

Does one 'repertorise' the juvenile nematodes in the centre, or the mature nematodes in the top right picture? All are useful, but the materia medica has concentrated upon naked-eye observations so anyone with functioning sense organs remains empowered to join in the work. If one can observe any implicated creatures this is a useful part of the description if you have the expertise.

(Photographic credits are on page 180)

(Continued from page 27)

action between, for instance, the Kali salts enable us to fine-tune the treatment. Thus, not only can the change in shape of the enzyme expose or obstruct the reaction site, it will do so and be the cause of some forms of disease.

Many of the biochemical activities of cells such as starch and protein production, photosynthesis, and respiration, fall within the class of oxidation-reduction processes. Some elements serve as structural components, such as calcium and silica. Calcium combines with pectic acid, to form the lamella in the plant cell wall. Silica gives the skeletal strength to a plant, as is found in the haulm and the skin of seeds. Phosphorus is found in the sugar phosphate chains of both DNA and RNA, but its function is by no means limited to providing the backbone of the genetic material. Backbone function is also found in the hardest parts of the plant, such as bark and cambium. Too much or too little phosphorus causes degeneration, a generative function as the word implies. Nitrogen is an essential component of amino-acids, chlorophyll and nucleotides. Sulphur is also found in amino-acids, thus forming a component of proteins.

Plant Structure and Tissues.

The plant body is 'upside down', the roots being the equivalent of the mouth, the stem is the backbone, while the leaves form the respiratory, digestive and urinary systems. Therefore, we begin at the bottom, just as in most materia medicas for humans the division begins at the head.

The Roots

The roots fulfil diverse functions, not the least of which is the anchoring of the plant. They also take up nutrients and water. They also anchor the topsoil, thus reducing erosion. Two other functions are storage and conduction. Most roots are important storage organs. Examples are the potato, the carrot, sugar beet and onion. The foods are manufactured above ground in photosynthesis and are transported through the phloem to the roots where they are stored. Sometimes the roots themselves are the food, but generally it is digested and the products of this process are channelled back through the xylem to the above ground parts to be processed again. The phloem and xylem form the capillary system, comparable to the circulation in humans.

In the biennials - plants that require two years to reach maturity - great quantities of food are stored in the roots in the first year. In the second year these are used to produce flowers and fruits or seeds. Water and nutrients are absorbed by the roots and move through the xylem to the leaves. Some hormones are produced in the roots, such as cytokinins and gibberellins, which are also transported upwards because they are needed for growth and development.

The different root systems can be classified easily. The primary root comes from the embryo of the seed. In some plants this becomes a taproot, growing vertically downward with lateral roots developing out of it. The older lateral roots are situated near the base of the root, where root and stem meet. The younger ones are found near the tip. This taproot system is found in dicots and gymnosperms. In monocots the primary root is short lived and additional roots form from the stem. These, together with the lateral roots form a fibrous root system. In such a system all roots are equally important. The extent of a root system is dependent on a variety of factors, which include moisture content of the soil, its temperature, and the composition of the soil. Some roots occupy a much larger space underground than the whole of the plant above ground. Alfalfa roots go to a depth of 6 meters or more. A 4 month old rye plant had roots which covered an area of 639 m^2, or 130 times the area of the above ground shoots. Yet the roots covered only 6 litres of soil.

During the growth cycle of a plant, it maintains a balance between synthesising surface to produce food, and the area needed for absorption of water and nutrients. Many roots grow continuously, only stopping at low temperatures or drought. The root always follows the path of least resistance, seeking spaces that earlier plant roots have created for it before they died and rotted. This has the further advantage of providing organic matter in which roots grow better. The root tip is covered by a cap, a mass of thimble-like cells which protect the stem behind it and helps to penetrate the soil. As it grows the root cap pushes forward while the cells in its periphery are sloughed off. These cells and the root tip are covered by a slimy sheath, the mucigel, which lubricates the root to provide easy passage. In disease this mucigel may be dry or extend over the whole root.

The most familiar type of root for food storage is probably the tuber as found in the potato. When grown from seed, the tubers form at the end of what is called the stolon. Cuttings of tubers used for propagation give rise to tubers found at the end of rhizomes. A bulb is a large bud with a small stem and many modified leaves around it. These leaves are like scales with thickened bases to store food, such as in the onion. Corms are superficially like bulbs but they consist of thick fleshy stem tissue, much smaller than bulbs. The food is stored within the corms of, for instance, the crocus, gladiolus, and cyclamen. Kohlrabi is an example of a plant using the thick fleshy above ground stem for food storage.

Stems

The primary tissues of stems have similar growth periods as the roots. The latter grow during the dark half of the moon while the former have their phase of growth during the light half, thus enabling the plant to grow evenly. The stem grows in a different manner than the root. Roots grow through cell division and elongation. The stem grows largely through internodal elongation. The stem grows as a more or less continuous hollow cylinder, as a cylinder of discrete strands, or as a system of strands scattered throughout the ground tissue The phloem is generally situated outside the xylem.

Leaves

In dicots the leaves have a blade and petiole; the blade is sometimes divided into leaflets. Stomata (pores) are generally more abundant on the upper surface. The mesophyll is a photosynthetic tissue permeated by airspace and veins. The latter are made by phloem and xylem, surrounded by a sheath called skin. The xylem is situated on the upper side and the phloem on the underside. Most monocots, which include grasses, have leaves made up of a blade and a sheath encircling the stem. The leaves of C3 and C4 grasses have different anatomical properties because they are adapted to the absorption of different carbon compounds. Shoots are a collective of stems and leaves that have physical and developmental associations. The capillary or vascular system will branch off in each node to provide the leaves with a connection through which starch and protein can be transported in either direction.

Photosynthesis

Photosynthesis is the process whereby light energy is converted into chemical energy, enabling carbon to be fixed into organic compounds, like starch and protein. The usual equation runs as follows: $CO_2 + 2H_2A + \text{light} >> (CH_2O) + H_2O + 2A$.

H_2A represents either water or another substance that can be oxidised (that is, from which electrons can be removed) and (CH_2O) represents carbohydrate.

The pigments that enable photosynthesis are chlorophyll and carotenoids, grouped in units called photosystems. Absorbed light turns their electrons to a higher energy level. Most of these organisms contain two photosystems. Not all reactions require light. Photosynthesis is a necessary process in plants to produce food and release oxygen, which is needed by nearly all living entities. Without photosynthesis the plant requires a symbiotic relationship with another organism that helps it in this process.

Flowers

The vegetative shoot is directly transformed into a reproductive apex. The flowers are either separated in sex, with male and female characteristics, or are hermaphrodite, meaning that both sexual functions are found in the same flower. The male characteristic is found in the stamen which produces pollen, the plant equivalent of semen. The female characteristic is found in the ovaries, which after pollination produce the seed, nut, or fruit.

How to Use the Remedies

When using homoeopathy, one is giving of a very small dose of a substance, possibly a poison, which in a large dose would cause similar symptoms to the illness presented for treatment. There is no strength to a homoeopathic preparation other than what is known as 'potency'. As opposed to conventional medicines or agricultural treatments, the potency is not determined by the gross amount of active substance present. Instead it is determined by the number of times it has been ground, diluted and shaken according to the homoeopathic method.

The remedies stimulate the organism's intrinsic defensive mechanism; once the initial dose has acted on the plant, a series of internal responses occur to re-establish the balance of vital forces within it. Homoeopathic treatments act as a trigger and, for this reason, do not usually need frequent re-application. In fact, over-use can counter the benefits achieved and in many cases can worsen the problem.

Application

You must always follow the application guidelines carefully. Homoeopathic remedies are easy to apply on both small plots and in commercial agriculture, but there are some basic rules that must be followed. Any liquid dispensing device can be used: watering can, backpack sprayer, boomspray, etc. It can be injected into reticulation systems at the tank or the pump. On large areas some calculation of watering rates may be necessary to administer the correct dose.

Do not mix homoeopathic medicine with anything other than water. Do not use commercial herbicides, pesticides, fungicides or fertilisers for at least 10 days after applying homoeopathic remedies. Quite simply this may counteract all the positive effect.

Excessively acidic or alkaline water may affect the remedy's action, usually just slowing it down. Make sure your spraying equipment is not contaminated. Residues of agricultural chemicals may antidote the remedy. If in doubt, rinse well with the hottest water possible, or steam clean.

Application rates

1st: 500ml/500l per hectare or 10ml/10l on small areas
2nd: 250ml/500l per hectare or 5ml/10l
3rd: 125ml/500l per hectare or 1ml/10l

Procedure

First put in the remedy, then add the water. This is usually sufficient for mixing evenly, Where this is impractical, for example in large tanks, spend a minute or two stirring it with a large stick.

The most important part: each homoeopathic remedy should be allowed to act before it is repeated. In the event of a worsening of the symptoms, usually visible within 48 hours, use the antidote as below.

Antidoting

If an adverse reaction is elicited by the remedy, look up the antidotes under the description of the remedy which you have applied, and use a single application. In case you do not have the antidote in your possession, apply the third application rate (see above) of the same remedy which you have used to bring out the effect.

Potency

It is recommended that the 6x potency is used.

Materia Medica

The *materia medica* is presented using the following template:

Name of the remedy as known in homoeopathy

Common name of the source - plant, mineral, element or animal

Latin name, where appropriate

Natural order (NO) - where the remedy is of plant or animal origin, sometimes including the Family

Symbol of element or chemical formula

Method of preparation of mother tincture (trituration or solution)

Clinical description, i.e. symptoms and/or pest and disease

General description, i.e. history of its use and indications

Appearance

Relations

It is recommended that after careful observation, relevant plant analysis and soil tests, the appropriate remedy is applied in the 6x potency. Always use a single application, to be repeated only when effects have been observed indicating that curative action has come to an end before completion. Some remedies carry an extra caution about repetition, not to be ignored. No responsibility is taken for wrong or repeated applications against these guidelines. Only trees and shrubs can be given repeated doses, but never more than 2 doses in a year, with intervals indicated by curative actions only.

Acetic Acid

Glacial acetic acid. CH_3COOH. Distilled water is used for attenuations 1x and 2x, very dilute spirit for 3x and 4x, rectified spirit for the 5x and higher.

CLINICAL
Weeds. Respiratory insufficiency, photosynthesis impaired. Chlorosis. Wilting.

GENERAL
The leading features of *Acet. acid* are excessive wasting and debility, presupposing a strong influence on plant life. In the crude form it has been used extensively on weeds, but its dangers to other plants must not be overlooked. Like all acids it can be used for weed control.

Weeds tell much about the state of the soil - its pH level, structure and nutrient content. It is advisable to let weeds grow for as long as possible before they set seed. Their eradication will return nutrients to the soil. Deep rooted weeds break up compacted soil and reduce water-logging.

Acetic acid plays an important role in the Krebs cycle which regulates respiration (Fuller and Ritchie, 1967.)

Acetic acid in the potencies will be effective in disturbances of the Krebs cycle.

Caution is written more largely over this remedy picture than any other remedy including the tissue salts. Application must be precise, with no spillage. The advantage of using the potencies is clear - no residues remain in the soil and no build-up of toxic levels is possible. It is advised to use this remedy pre-planting or seeding.

Acetic acid can be conceived of as an 'organ remedy' of the first order. Together with the *Oxalic acid* and the *Citric acid* this trio forms the key to respiratory and photosynthesis disorders.

RELATIONS
Compare: *Citric acid, Oxalic acid.*

Aconitum Napellus

Monk's hood. NO *Compositae*. Tincture of the whole plant.

CLINICAL
Stripe rust, leaf rust, beet roots, bean rust, marigold rust, iris rust, poplar, rose, snapdragon. Banana rust. Bean blossom thrips. Rust mite. Active congestion of the capillary system. Rust - rapid onset of symptoms. Worse cold dry nights, injury, mechanical damage. Barley yellow dwarf virus.

GENERAL
Grows in moist pastures and waste places in mountainous districts. The rapidity of action determines its appropriateness for conditions where symptoms set in with great intensity, as in rust. *Aconite* is homoeopathic to tension. Active congestion of the capillary system, especially after cold spells, cold dry air at night. The keen cutting winds of the hills (amongst which the plant grows) give the signature of its remedial action. Chill, injury or mechanical damage. Extreme sensitivity to light. Plants have a marked thirst. Great and sudden sinking of strength, both effects of heat and cold. This remedy has been used with great success in the treatment of rusts.

APPEARANCE
Rust with bright red colouring and yellow margins. Hard red swellings of the leaves, bloated and hot and bright red. Red spots, swollen and shiny and broad. Sudden wilting.

Yellow dwarf virus - Wheat:
Interveinal chlorosis is the first sign of the yellow dwarf. The colour is yellow/orange and there is less pronounced reddening of leaf tips.

Yellow dwarf virus - Barley:
Barley has a bright yellowing of the leaves and pale yellow interveinal chlorosis. Sometimes reddening of the leaf tips occurs. In all cases of yellow dwarf, if infection occurs in young plants, they stunt and grain yields are sharply reduced, often with shrivelling of the grains. In general sick plants are stimulated to produce seed to ensure survival of the species. In grain, tillering is poorly developed and sterile heads are common. (McKirdy and Jones, 1993. Loughman, 1994.)

Yellow dwarf virus - Grasses:
Grasses do not always show symptoms. Phalaris shows yellowing, whereas the rye grasses show reddening or purpling of the leaf tips. The latter should be treated with *Belladonna*.

Epidemics appear to follow every 2-3 years. It is restricted to high rainfall areas. Yield losses can run up to 80% in cereals. Late infection can reduce the yield up to 20%. There is no chemical control for yellow dwarf after infection. The only available control is killing the aphid vector when detected (Grain development Corporation, 1994). But if the infection has already started, the plants are lost. *Aconite* and *Belladonna* can do much for this problem even after infection.

It is estimated, that there are many hundreds of fungi associated with rusts. They cause a yellowish small patch or spot on the upper surface of the leaves. That develops into a powdery pustule, the powder being the stalks which produce the spores. These stalks rupture the epidermis, which is why they appear raised above the surface. Wind or rain and water sprinklers spread the spores.

In conventional agriculture, rust control is very difficult because the spores can be blown or washed over large areas very quickly. Some rusts cause galls which are uniform in appearance and connected with particular fungi. The economics of spraying rusts with chemicals are prohibitive on wheat and other grains (Grain Development Corporation, 1994). Rusts are also used on certain weeds as biological control - examples are skeleton weed and blackberry. Some rusts need two hosts in areas with cold winters and snow. Barberry is the second host for wheat rusts. Poplar rust spends the winter on the larch.

FLOWERS AND FRUITS
Flowers dry, hot, overproduction of pollen, slowing the setting of fruit.

WATERING
Thirsty, but generally worse watering.

RELATIONS
Compare: *Ammonium preps, Belladonna*
Antidote: *Belladonna*

Allium Cepa

Common red onion. NO *Liliacea*. Tincture of the onion, or of the whole fresh plant. Gathered from July to August.

CLINICAL
Gangrene, apple scab, downy and powdery mildew on gooseberries and cucumbers. Respiratory problems. No uptake of nutrients. Onion fly and carrot fly. Good companion to carrots. Rabbits, mice and rats. Weevils, mites, late blight on tomatoes and potatoes. Brown rot stone fruit. Potassium problems, helps roses. Scales, aphids, thrips, mites.

GENERAL
Allium will cure inflammations and increased secretions as in apple scab, downy and powdery mildews. Wounds, after damage, that do not heal. Not to be used on beans and peas, as it inhibits their growth. This is confirmed in the potencies.

The roots of the plants have a bad smell. The plants are thirsty and seem to crave nutrients and fertiliser. Evaporation is increased or totally absent. Photosynthesis is impaired, respiration is diminished (oxygen meter at night to check), consequent development of mildews. Gangrenous spots.

APPEARANCE
Leaves droop, covered in mildews, fruits may also be affected.

WATER NEEDS
High.

WARNING
Do not use on antagonistic plants such as beans and peas!

Ammonium Carbonicum

Sesqui carbonate of ammonia, Sal volatile. $[(NH_4)_2CO_3]CO_2$ solution, distilled in water.

CLINICAL
Capillary engorgement, photosynthesis defective. Roots dark red with orange surrounds. Stem rusts, stripe rust, leaf rust, aphids, banana rust thrips.

GENERAL
A condition of under oxygenation. Plants are greatly affected by cold air, wet, stormy weather and rain. They pick up when weather gets warmer. Capillary engorgement results in sap loss. Flowers are premature, photosynthesis defective. Chlorophyll deficiency as in chlorosis, reduces the capacity to incorporate simple molecules into complex compounds such as starch. Chlorosis is the lack of pigment giving the leaves a pale green or yellow colour.

Lack of chlorophyll induces the plant to shed leaves since it cannot afford to expend food on leaves that do not function. In deciduous trees this happens every autumn and the tree goes dormant during the winter. In other plants, chlorosis indicates disease such as blotch barley yellow dwarf virus, stripe, rust, halo-spot, spot blotch, yellow spot and nutrition imbalance such as manganese, zinc or iron deficiency. When *Ammonium* is indicated, there are many symptoms. The roots are usually dry, sometimes showing vesicles or swellings. The plant usually requires frequent watering, but nutrients are not absorbed, thus adding to the difficulties of photosynthesis. Respiration is particularly difficult. Nitrogen fixation in beans and peas may be affected by a molybdenum deficiency.

When excess ammonium is applied it turns to nitrogenous nutrient. This in turn fixes sulphur, or in other words it antidotes, or is inimical. Sulphur then becomes deficient in the plant. Ammonium sulphate is indicated in such problems as it will modify the nitrogenous action and augment the action of the sulphur component. The relationship between nitrogen and sulphur is important in the diseases and symptoms that are produced when either is excessive or deficient. (Spencer et al. 1977.)

The rusts are dark red as in *Belladonna*. The flowers appear premature, and pollinate heavily or not at all. The female parts do not function properly and fruit setting is incomplete due to this.

APPEARANCE
The rust manifests itself as pustules full of dark, reddish brown powdery spores on stems and leaves (both sides), sheaths and heads. The spores fall off easily, the pustules are oval and elongated. Surrounding leaf or stem surfaces are usually

ruptured. Towards the end of the season, as the plant matures, the pustules produce black spores. Wheat stem rust also affects barley, durum and triticale. The fungus survives on green hosts such as grasses.

Rust assumes epidemic proportions when summer/autumn rains allow wheat or barley to survive throughout summer. This disease can cause record crop loss within very short time at the end of a season. Warm (15-30 degrees Celsius) and humid conditions favour this disease. There are resistant varieties, but rust is versatile and develops new strains to survive. There are no chemical treatments for seed, and foliar spray is very costly. *Ammonium carbonica* or *Belladonna* will quickly put an end to rust infection. Spraying is done early in the season (cf *Aconite*).

FLOWERS AND FRUITS

Rust also attacks heads, thus making flowering problematic, and fruit setting nigh impossible, resulting in total crop loss over a short period. Critical nitrate to nitrogen levels in the petioles of pumpkin at early fruiting lie at 4,000 mg/kg for irrigated and 8,000 - 8,400 mg/kg for dryland crops. (Swaider et al. 1988.)

WATER NEEDS

High.

RELATIONS

Antidote to: *Sulphur, Sulphuric acid, Molybdenum.*
Compare: *Ammonium sulphate, Nitric acid, Kali Nitricum.*
See also: *Phosphorus, Kali* preps, *Calcarea* preps, *Magnesia* preps, *Ferrum* preps, *Manganum, Cuprum, Zinc, Natrum* preps. *Ammonium* affects all these when in excess.
Complementary: *Molybdenum.*

Ammonium Muriaticum

Ammonium chloride. Sal ammoniac.. NH_4Cl. Solution.

CLINICAL
Defective photosynthesis. Capillary system engorged; decomposition of sap. Slimy rots, wet rots, stem rot. Ergot, early stages. Lodging.

GENERAL
Ammonium muriaticum is less sensitive to cold weather than *Ammonium carbonicum* The capillary system collapses in rots causing the plants to lodge. The flowers produce a sticky slime as in ergot, and *Ammonium muriaticum* might prove to be a possible remedy for ergot. From the available information, this would only be applicable in the early stages. Photosynthesis is impaired with consequent low protein levels. Eruptions on the leaves like blotch.

As *Ammonium muriaticum* is the chief constituent of nitrogen, it is self-evident that in all cases where nitrate or nitrite is abundant in plants, it will cause problems. Cankers and rots, mainly wet rots, are the consequence. Nitrogen, as stated elsewhere, makes the plant obese; bloated and watery as it is, it invites all sorts of bacteria and fungi to restore that balance so upset by chemical fertilisers.

Ammonium produces in toxicity a form of rots as well as photosynthesis deficiency. Hahnemann considered the triturations to be more active than the solutions, because they are said to be more stable.

Ammonium carbonicum is considered by Leeser to be of better service. He considers the hydroxides to be unsuitable for therapeutic purposes. (Leeser, 1936.)

In the same way, if a human eats junk food, disease is the result. NPK is junk food for plants, the consequences of which are numerous pests and diseases. A study at the University of Kentucky has shown that excess plant nitrogen attracts aphids. USDA tests have proven that spider mites lay an average of 5.4 eggs per day. High levels of nitrogen increase this to 10 and more per day. (Hylton, 1974.) High nitrogen levels also cause fruit drop in tomato.

Nitrogen causes a rise in amino acids which in turn attracts pests. A Temple University test showed that aphids prefer plants with high amino acid content. Nitrogen is, together with potassium, antagonistic to boron, thus leading to boron deficiency and the consequent crown rot, sickle leaf and hollow stem in turnip and cauliflower. Over-liming can also stop boron uptake. If all three are present, as is quite often the case, celery will have short cracked stems, broccoli will have brownish groups of dry buds on the heads, beetroot will have black spot and cracks on the inside, carrots show yellowing of the margins of the leaves, whilst young leaves will suffer from die back. This may happen when boron is at less that one part per million in the soil. Thus the potency here is the important thing.

Hahnemann spoke of the "dynamis" as the active principle; thus, a 6x potency is one part per million and acts as a dynamic trigger, because of its division and succusion, the latter being the main difference between a solution and a potency.

APPEARANCE
As ergot, rots, and blotch are described elsewhere, we will refrain from unnecessary repetition.

WATER NEEDS
High.

RELATIONS
Antidote to: *Cuprum, Cuprum sulphuricum, Sulphur, Sulphuric acid, Molybdenum.*
See also: *Ammonium carbonicum.*
Complementary: *Phosphorus, Kali, Boron, Calcarea, Magnesia, Manganese, Ferrum, Cuprum, Zinc and the Natrum* salts, *Molybdenum.*
Inimical: *Boron.*

Aranea Diadema

The papal cross spider. NO Arachidna. Tincture of live insect.

CLINICAL
Most pests that are prey to web weaving spiders.

GENERAL
Grauvogl is the main authority on *Aranea*. He says that it is of the hydrogenoid constitution. By this he meant, translated for plants, abnormal sensitivity to cold and damp weather, worse from rain and waterlogging or damp cold winds. In such conditions plants become weak and prone to pest attack. To date, no specifications can be given on the pests that can be controlled with this remedy, but from what is known from the spider's food habit, it will take locusts, flies, butterflies, moths and practically everything else that flies in its web. *Mygale*, *Tarantula and Theridion* species should be compared. Orb weavers cannot afford to be selective in the choice of prey and their poisons, although considered not as potent as those of hunting spiders who can choose their prey, may have a wider range of action.

RELATIONS
Compare: *Mygale, Tarantula, Theridion*.

Arnica Montana

Leopards bane. NO Compositae. Tincture of whole fresh plant.

CLINICAL
After transplants or pruning. Do not use on open wounds. Plants both transplanted and pruned cannot be given *Arnica*. These should be treated with *Calendula*.

GENERAL
Grows in the Alps and other mountains. *Arnica* is a first aid remedy par excellence; trauma in all forms and varieties, pests, pruning. Transplants and mechanical injury will be met by *Arnica* as by no other remedy. *Arnica* may not be sprayed onto open wounds as it will cause inflammation and suppuration. *Arnica* has been used extensively for the indications with good results.

Tumors on trees as a result of wrong pruning, even cancerous growths can be healed, provided they are the result of some form of injury. Root damage after transplants, after hail, when damaged leaves become yellow, or red as in deciduous trees in autumn.

APPEARANCE
Wilting after transplants due to root damage; mist *Arnica* onto the leaves. Weeping wounds after pruning. Water *Arnica* in on the roots. Rotting grafts, tumors on old wounds, especially on large trees where large limbs leave big scars. Scar tissue soft and spongy with rotting pulp underneath. Swellings hot, hard, shiny, red, bluish or yellow spots. Yellow spots caused by bruises or disease, eruption of small raised spots as in yellow rust.

WATER NEEDS
Thirsty when wilting from transplants. Otherwise little above normal.

RELATIONS
Compare: *Calendula, Ferrum, Carbo vegetabilis*.

Belladonna

Deadly nightshade. *Atropa belladonna*. NO Solanacea. Tincture of whole plant when beginning to flower.

CLINICAL
Carnation rust, fuschia rust, iris rust, peach rust, raspberry rust. Rust with orange margins, darker red than *Aconite* worse cold damp weather. (Cold and dry; *Aconite.*) Barley yellow dwarf virus, white florets, where other colour is healthy. Take-all, anthracnose. Acacia spotting bug. Banana rust thrips, rust mite.

GENERAL
Grows in dry soil on the slopes of hills. Goats and rabbits can eat nightshade with impunity. Cats and dogs are only mildly affected. In plants, it has been used with very good results on rust in fruit trees. *Belladonna* acts on all parts of the organism. Sensitivity to light (*Aconite*) is a leading feature, making for leaves that either do not open, or burn. Sensitivity to changes from warm to cold in damp weather, and draughts of air.

Belladonna, like *Aconite*, is fast acting; consequently for symptoms that develop rapidly. Heat, redness and burning. Darker red than *Aconite.* Red with orange margins (*Aconite* red and yellow). Purple red, orangey yellow. Red parts such as flowers and fruit look pale. Blistering from heat. Swelling and bluish redness. Sunburn. Windburn. *Belladonna* has been used for the dark rusts with excellent results.

There are hundreds of different fungi that are supposed to cause the diseases we call rust. Generally they cause some sort of small yellow or red patch or spot on the surface of leaves. Under each spot, on the lower surface of the leaf, a powdery pustule appears. This happens when the fungus produces the stalks of spores. These stalks burst the epidermis of the leaf, and the spores are then blown away in the wind.

Rusts are, in general, difficult to control because new infections can occur over a large area. Rusts develop very quickly. Hence *Aconite* and *Belladonna* as rapidly acting remedies can do much to control this.

Some rusts stimulate plant cells to form galls. Rust in cereal crops cannot easily be sprayed economically with conventional methods. *Aconite* and *Belladonna* can do this satisfactorily.

Some rusts need two different host species to complete their life cycle and survive the cold in areas with cold winters. For example, in Europe, the poplar rust spends part of its life on the larch, while wheat rust spends part of its life on barberry. They produce thick walled spores in autumn. These survive the winter to infect the next sequential species in the spring. Spore germination requires some moisture, but in general, little can be said about weather conditions that favour rust disease.

Fuchsia rust (*Pucciniastrum epilobii*) causes purple-red blotches on the upper leaf surface. These blotches subsequently die and become dry and brittle, with purple spores on the edges on the edges on the underside of the leaves. The spores can range from yellow to orange-red or purple.

Iris rust (*Puccinia irides*) is characterised by rusty red powdery spots on both sides of the leaves. The leaves turn chlorotic around the spots, which can spread to the whole leaf. Although the plant may lose some leaves from this rust, it generally survives. This rust is spread mainly by wind and it is worse in warm and humid weather. Irises grown both from rhizomes and bulbs are affected, the former more than the latter.

Barley yellow dwarf virus affects many species of the Graminacae. All cereals and many grasses fall prey to it. It only survives in living plants. Infection is restricted to the phloem. The virus can only be seen with the electron microscope.

Aphids carry the virus from plant to plant. An aphid needs to feed on an infected plant to become a lifelong carrier. (McKirdy and Jones, 1993.)

Four different types of yellow dwarf virus have been identified. Their differences are expressed in their vectors (different species of aphids), their transmitability and the damage extent.

Two types of aphid, the oat (*Rhopalosiphum padi*) and corn leaf aphid (*Rhopalosiphum maidis*), are the main species to spread yellow dwarf. The oat aphid feeds on oat, wheat, barley and grasses. Cornleaf aphids feed on cornleaf barley and some grasses. Three more aphid species have been connected with its spread. The grain aphid (*Sitobion spp.*) and two cereal root aphids (*Rhopalosiphum insertum* and *Rhopalosiphum rufiabdominalis*).

Aphids migrate in autumn and spring from kikuyu grass, paspalum, couch and African lovegrass. Kikuyu seems to be more infected than others. (McKirdy and Jones, 1993. Loughman, 1994.)

APPEARANCE
Symptoms are often confused with nutrient deficiencies, waterlogging and other stresses. The leaf symptoms differ between oat, barley and wheat.

Oat is more prominent in the crimson pink reddening of the leaves, reason it is included under *Belladonna*. From the tip down the leaf blotches, turning red on older leaves, while the younger, shows the interveinal chlorosis. The varieties that turn yellow/orange should be treated with *Aconite*.

Red spots, rust, sometimes oozing sap, red, purple or bluish. Swelling of eruptions. Rust with orange or dark yellow margins. Dark brown spots. Roots shiny and swollen or dry and swollen. Gangrenous parts of stems, leaves and flowers. Red spots the colour of blood.

FLOWERS AND FRUITS
Flowers are deficient in pollen (*Aconite* opposite). Small fruits, falling prematurely. Leaves falling due to rust. Scarlet redness of rust on leaves, stems and flowers. Red spots on fruits.

RELATIONS
Compare: *Aconite, Ammonium.*

Berberis

Common barberry. NO Berberidacea. Tincture of the bark of the root.

CLINICAL
Rust, mildew.

GENERAL
Grows on hedges throughout Britain. According to Prof. Henslow, "it was thought by farmers in the middle of the last (19th) century, that barberry blighted wheat if it grew near the hedge. Botanists thought the idea ridiculous, yet the farmers are right. Their observations consisted of the occurrence of rust in the wheat grown closely to barberry, which extended steadily across the whole crop.

"A fungus attacks the leaves of barberry, producing orange coloured spots. Its spores attack the wheat. These develop parasitic threads within the leaf, from which arise the red rust spores. Following this, dark brown or black spores consisting of two cells, called wheat mildew, appear. After some time these form one celled red spores, which attack the barberry and the cycle is completed. Barberry is the primary host plant of this cycle." (Henslow, quoted by Clarke.)

The roots are affected in a peculiar manner producing whitish vesicles on the epidermis. The roots feel dry to the touch, or are covered in a frothy viscid slime. The vesicles may appear red as in rust, while the whitish froth is connected with mildew.

The plant is either very thirsty or requires little water. Nutrients are either taken up very rapidly or not at all. The evaporation rate is higher than normal which accounts for thirsty plants. Respiration and photosynthesis impaired, due to mildew or rust. The plant has a tendency to lodging.

Flowers have incomplete stamen or produce no pollen. The ovaries may not function properly resulting in impaired fruit-setting capacity.

The rust is small, pustular, red, which gradually turns brownish and larger.

RELATIONS
Compare: *Aconite, Ammonium, Belladonna.*

Bombyx

Procession caterpillar. *Bombyx processiona*. NO *Lepidoptera*. Tincture of the live caterpillars.

CLINICAL
Caterpillars, vegetable loopers, sawfly larvae, army-worms, cabbage moths and other caterpillars.

GENERAL
The true bombyx is not a very large caterpillar and is today known as the white cedar moth, *Leptocneria reducta*. It is about 45 mm long, dark brown, with yellow head and masses of long grey and black hairs which cause skin irritation on contact.

Clarke mentions that: "...in one case a boy shook a large number of caterpillars from a tree on his naked chest. It caused an itching so severe, that he had to run for assistance. Then fever, somnolency, delirium and finally death ensued." (Clarke, 1991.)

The caterpillars live in colonies at the base of the tree during the day and feed on the foliage at night. After denuding the tree they walk in a single file to the next, which behaviour accounts for the name. They produce two generations per year.

Rodale's periodical relates the case of a commercial peanut and soybean farmer (1976). He prepared a crude product from vegetable loopers. Control was very successful. Another report from 1978 mentioned sawfly larvae being used in a similar fashion.

Bombyx in potency has been used to treat most caterpillars on most crops as a generic remedy. Both as a spray and in the trickle system it is effective. In both cases the plants become immune to caterpillar infestations.

RELATIONS
Compare: *Cantharis, Sambucus niger, Valeriana, Vibernum.*

Borax

Borax veneta. Natrum biboraticum, $Na_2B_4O_7$ - Trituration and solution.

CLINICAL
Boron imbalances.

GENERAL
Boron stands at the head of Group 3 in the table of Mendelieff. The fact that boron is called a micro-nutrient is because a minimal quantity is necessary for plants compared to the total amount of each of the other elements and the aggregate of all the nutrients. Due to its apparent insignificant position it has been overlooked until recent times.

However the micro-nutrients, precisely due to their minimal presence, form a very important part of plant life. The so-called 'plant-foods', nitrogen, phosphorus and potassium (NPK), although important, merely support its daily maintenance. A plant can live for a relatively long period without too much of these macro-nutrients, while the inability to take up the micro-elements will result in severe symptoms in a relatively short time, establishing serious disease.

Like *Aluminium* and *Alumen*, with which *Borax* has a close relationship on account of its belonging in the same group, the symptoms of *Borax* are clear cut. The bulk of the symptoms come from toxicity reports from the agricultural departments.

Toxicity with boron was not recognised till 1985. Before that time it was confused with netblotch, a fungal disease. In grains only barley appears to suffer from boron toxicity, as other grains have not yielded any symptoms.

Boron toxicity shows up in different plant families with slightly different symptoms. On grains it resembles netblotch. The symptoms appear as dark brown spots on the edges and tip of the leaf blade which turn necrotic. In netblotch the spots do not enlarge, but in boron toxicity they become so large and numerous that the leaves die. Moreover, netblotch is surrounded by a chlorotic halo, whereas boron toxicity is not. (Khan et al. 1985.)

On cassavas it looks like symptoms of aluminium toxicity. The development follows a particular pattern of yellow to white spots, mainly along the leaf margins towards the tip. These are surrounded by a dark halo, become necrotic and give the leaves a jagged edge. Boron excess stunts growth and can also produce a diffused chlorosis, beginning at the tip of senescent leaves. Plants may recover later in life. Boron toxicity occurs on highly alkaline soils, as opposed to aluminium toxicity which is dependent on high acidity. (Khan et al. 1985.)

Boron deficiency also causes stunted growth (dwarfing) and slight chlorosis. Plants recover quickly without reduction in size and yield. (Krochmal and Samuels, 1968.)

Bovista

Warted puffball. *Lycoperdon bovista*. NO Fungi. Trituration.

CLINICAL
Spider mite. Ovarian problems such as deformation. Capillary relaxation. Moist and dry rots. Moulds.

GENERAL
"This globular fungus which, according to reports, is eaten in Italy before it is ripe, becomes filled while ripening with the blackish dust that breaks the husk which contains it with a slight noise." (Clarke, 1991.)

The signature points to bloatedness, puffiness and enlargement. Ovarian problems in flowers. Moist and dry rots in many plants. Root rots with putrid smell. Plants are thirsty, more so in the afternoon and evening.

The spider mite can just be seen by the unaided eye, mainly because of its contrasting colour. The females are present in greater numbers and are harder to spot because they are pale green. In winter the females turn orange-red, but hide under the bark in the junction of branches or at the base of the plants. In spring they feed on the young shoots or seedlings, turn green again, and move back up the plant.

Bean debris harbours those that overwinter. In hot dry weather they do the most damage. Heavy rain reduces their numbers. The damage is visible as chlorosis, drying out and becoming brittle. Leaves turn grey.

Bovista was tried for fairy ring spot on turf but proved to be a failure. In the process its action on the spider mite was a welcome and happy result.

Calcarea Carbonica

Impure calcium carbonate. $CaCO_3$. Trituration of the middle layer of oyster shells or carbonate of lime (Hahnemann and Koch).

CLINICAL
Calcium deficiency as in bitter pit in apples, calcium excess on calcium rich soils. Plants obese with lax fibre, pale, chalky look in stems and leaves. Damping off. Nitrogen excess. Anthracnose. Thrips.

GENERAL
"*Calcarea* is one of the great monuments of the genius of Hahnemann. His method of preparing insoluble substances brought to light in this instance a whole world of therapeutic power, formerly unknown." (Clarke, 1991.) It is essential to have an intimate acquaintance with the Calcium preparations as they are pivotal to the understanding of homoeopathy as a whole, and its application in agriculture in particular. *Calcarea* preparations have a wide range and a deep action. Handle with care is not an unnecessary precaution. Too much dosing can set up severe aggravation in the crop and it is difficult to counteract it, as *Calcarea carbonica* is an important constituent in the plant body. Calcium, being a building block in plants, has a consequent low mobility. (Epstein, 1972.)

Cassava spp. root systems are very sensitive to calcium deficiency. (Forno et al. 1976.) Without sufficient calcium growth of the root is severely restricted, resulting in necrosis and decomposition. Above ground the leaves will burn and curl upwards at the tip although this is not always observed. (See also *Alumina* and *Alumen*) The leguminosa are more prone to show symptoms. (Edwards et al. 1977. Edwards and Kang, 1978.)

Excessive liming can induce deficiencies of potassium, manganese, magnesium, iron, copper or zinc. Treatment with calcium usually does not have any bearing on the yields of pasture, however it is a suitable carrier for both phosphorus and sulphur. (McLachlan and Norman, 1962.)

As Teste remarks in his materia medica: " I know that carbonate of lime, phosphorous, phosphoric acid and all other substances which enter largely into the composition of the human body, exercise a deep and pervasive action on the organism; but this is, it strikes me, an additional reason why it should not be administered at random." (Teste, 1991.)

Calcarea carbonica is closely related to *Belladonna* of which it is the "chronic". Repeated occurrence of rust in cereal crops may point to either calcium deficiency or excess in the soil. Demands for more irrigation is another indication for *Calcarea carbonica*.

In highly calcareous soils as found in the arid areas of the world, potassium applications can increase the yield in sugar beet by up to 79%. Micro-nutrients give better results when applied separately. (Kanch et al. 1990.)

Calcium- and magnesium-saturated soils severely depress potassium uptake regardless of the amount of potassium applied. (Anilkumar et al. 1989.) *Calcarea carbonica* is worse cold and better from heat. It corresponds to plants that are force-fed NPK resulting in obesity, sluggish capillaries and lax fibre. Large features, pale chalky look and feel in stems and leaves. Rather bloated than solid. *Calcarea carbonica* has been used both on acid and alkaline soils. The latter proved more successful than the former.

APPEARANCE

Growth is irregular. Late starters. Weaker in cold weather and rainy storms. Damping off in cereals and turf. Plants will look pale and collapse. Over-seeding will produce wrinkled, twisted, and distorted plants. Roots short and brown. Heavy use of nitrogen fertilisers creates soft turf and cereals which are more susceptible to attack. Nitrogen applied during establishment stage leads to sudden collapse of seedlings. Avoid watering late in the day so that soil is dry at night.

In calcium deficiency the growing tips die at the 2-4 leaf stage. Older plants show gradual capillary collapse, beginning at the leaf tips of the youngest leaves. Mottling of older leaves, folding backwards. Veins and edges remain green. Interveinal areas turn yellow-brown. Collapse of the flowering stalk; flowers wither and die. The leaves turn chlorotic and die. The under side of the leaves are pink in the interveinal spaces. (Mason and Gartrell, undated.)

When the soil is rich in calcium, as in the south west of Western Australia, many species of plants do not thrive. Limestone sands are too alkaline for many species. An acid manure such as chicken or pig manure can bring pH levels to normal. *Calcarea carbonica* will greatly benefit plants that have difficulty in alkaline soils, however, it is ecologically unsound practice to grow plants unsuitable to this soil type.

Sometimes potting mix is so acidic that transplants cause calcium shock. *Calcarea carbonica* can work miracles in such cases. *Calcarea carbonica* must not, however, be used indiscriminately because severe reactions can cause complete crop loss. Caution is written in bold type over the *Calcarea carbonica* picture. Deep acting elementary remedies like the Calcarea preparations require careful observation, frugal application, and close monitoring. By closely following instructions for application it can do wonders for plants that do not thrive. In annuals like cereals, one dose in the entire life-cycle of the crop is the maximum allowed. In trees, no more than once per year, with a maximum of three applications in a row. In shrubs, once per 2-3 years, and no more than three times in total.

In calcium rich or deficient soils it may be given when symptoms present themselves, or return after an interval.

APPEARANCE
Red margins on leaves, leaves yellow, sometimes swollen. Pale chalky Flowers too early, premature. Sterility of seed in fruit crops. Fruits do not set or mature. Spongy feel in seeds and fruits. No firmness, plant appears bloated, obese.

MICROSCOPIC
Obese cells, thin cell walls, accumulation of salts, high water content.

CHEMICAL
Excess water and nitrogen. Reduced protein levels.

FLOWERS AND FRUITS
Reduced flowering period. Flowers do not last. Premature fruit dropping, sterility, little or no seed or fruit. Fruits do not mature, small, shrivelled.

WATER NEEDS
Very thirsty, wilts easily when internal water is used up during dry spells.

RELATIONS
Antidote to: *Manganum*, Magnesia preps., Kali preps, Ferrum preps, *Cuprum, Zinc.*
Complementary: *Phosphorus, Sulphur, Sulphuricum acidum.*
Inimical: Kali, *Phosphorus* sometimes, but not in *Calcarea phosphoricum*, Magnesia preps, *Manganum, Ferrum, Cuprum, Zinc.*
Antidoted by: *Sulphur* but not in *Calcarea sulphurica.*

Calcarea Fluorata

Fluor spar. CaF_2. Trituration.

CLINICAL
Symptoms on the stems, trunks and twigs. Hard swollen nodes. Stem rot, spot blotch, stem end rot in avocado, stem nematode.

GENERAL
Calcarea fluorata is Schuessler's "bone salt". It is found at the surfaces of bones, the enamel in teeth, in elastic fibres and the cells of the epidermis. These latter have significance in plant use. Induration threatening suppuration. Spot blotch, stem rot and stem nematode. The skin or bark is dry and harsh.

APPEARANCE
Stem nematode (Meloidogyne spp.): Bases of plants swollen. Tillers may be distorted, stunted, and more numerous than healthy plants. The nematode causes a brown rot at the base of the plants which tend to die prematurely.

Spot blotch (Septoria spp.): Dark brown oblong spots or lesions on leaves and sheaths, often with yellow surrounds. Stem nodes infected with rot. This disease can lead to black point.

Stem rot (Dothiorella spp.): The fungus causing this disease lives on dead twigs and leaves. Spores are splashed onto fruit in rainy weather. Spores remain dormant until the fruit is ripening. A dark brown to black rot begins at stem end and gradually progresses down the fruit.

FLOWERS AND FRUITS
Barley florets die, black point symptoms on grain, rot on avocados.

RELATIONS
Antidote to: Ferrum, Magnesia, Manganum, Zinc.
Inimical: Magnesia, Phosphorus.
Antidoted by: Sulphur.
Complementary: Phosphorus, Sulphur.

Calcarea Phosphorica

Phosphate of lime. $Ca_3(PO_4)_2$. Trituration.

CLINICAL
Debility. Straggly, thin plants. Small fruits with soft skin, prone to rot. Stem rot, stem nematode, spot blotch, seed gall nematode, eye spot, tan spot, downy mildew. Mainly found in cereals.

GENERAL
Calcarea phosphorica has strong resemblance to *calcarea carbonica* but is by no means the same. Plants are straggly and thin, rather than fat and obese. They appear less chalky. The paleness is dirty-brownish *calcarea phosphorus* is more brittle than *Calcarea carbonica*. The epidermis is soft and thin and it cracks. The leaves are thin and brittle. The flowers are strongly affected: long stamen with abundant pollen yet small. Fruits, prone to rot, with soft skins. *Calcarea phosphorica* plants are sensitive to cold and damp weather. Leaves that show spots and eruptions, as is evident from the clinical section.

APPEARANCE
Net blotch. Develops first as small circular to elliptical dark brown spots which elongate and produce fine dark brown streaks along and across leaves, creating a distinct net-like pattern. When severe, it also affects the heads. The affected area turns yellow. Withering. Residue can produce spores over 2 years. Infection requires moist conditions, 15^0-25^0 C. Very humid conditions infect the seed.

Seed gall nematode (Meloidogyne spp.): wrinkled twisted or rolled leaves, stems swell at ground level. At heading, plants appear stunted and slow to mature. Instead of grain, there are hard brown/black seed galls. Affected heads are small. The nematode can survive in soil for two years. They are released from the gall in moist conditions, migrating in water films on leaves and sheaths, reaching immature heads. They enter immature florets, mate, reproduce and form galls.

Eye spot: (Cercosporella herpotrichoides) Lodging. Plants fall in all directions, breaking within two inches of the surface. Sooty mould on the break and under the sheaths. Brown or honey coloured lesions. Spores survive on residue, are spread by rain splash, and prefer moist conditions and 10^0C. Soil nitrogen levels are high.

Tan spot: (Cercosporella spp): Tan spots, yellow margins, leaves dry out and wither. It survives on stubble with small black fruiting bodies that release spores in wet conditions. The longer the wet period, the more severe the infection. Durum wheat, triticale and grasses. Not often seen in rye, barley or oats.

Downy mildew (Peronospora spp.): Young plants show leaf yellowing and severe stunting and excessive tillering. Many plants die at this stage. Older plants have thickened leathery leaves, twisted, fleshy and distorted heads (crazy top). Affected tillers produce no grain. Worse in moist conditions. It affects wheat, barley, oats, rye, durum and triticale, maize, sorghum and many grasses.

FLOWERS AND FRUITS
Flowers are severely affected, little or no grains. Flowers with long stamen and abundant pollen, fruit grains have soft skins and are prone to rot.

WATER NEEDS
Usually only occurs if water is too abundant.

The combined effect of calcium and phosphorus can be seen operating in this remedy; the epidermis is weak, making for many lesions in the form of spots and rots. The reproductive organs are severely affected so that crop losses occur. A single application during the lifetime of cereals is sufficient to arrest most problems.

CAUTIONS
As with all Calcium preparations, caution is important. Deep acting remedies that form part of the body of plants must never be over used or the negative effects will compound the existing problem.

RELATIONS:
Antidote to *Ferrum, Magnesia, Manganum, Zinc.*
Inimical: *Magnesia.*
Antidoted by : *Sulphur.*
Complementary: *Phosphorus, Sulphur.*

Calendula

Marigold. Calendula officinalis. NO Compositae. Tincture of the flowers or tincture of the whole plant.

CLINICAL
Transplants, pruning, storm or mechanical damage. Asparagus beetle, nematodes.

GENERAL
What *Arnica* is to trauma, *Calendula* is to open wounds. Where *Arnica* is of little or no use, or even dangerous to plants, *Calendula* comes to the rescue. It belongs in the same order of Compositae as *Arnica*. Lacerated and ulcerating wounds such as those found on roots that have been ripped or cut during transplants. *Calendula* will be of much help here, as confirmed in the field tests.

Calendula is antiseptic and restores vitality to the injured parts. It stops the entry of external opportunistic infections, as well as the proliferation of internal dormant viruses, but only in wounded plants. Nematodes cause these types of wounds. *Calendula* proved to be effective.

Arnica irritates, whilst *Calendula* soothes. Suitable for all cases where skin or bark is broken. Flowers of marigolds close when dark clouds pass overhead, therefore affected plants are usually worse in cloudy weather and during cold winter nights, which may be the cause of ulceration of pruning wounds or broken roots.

Calendula contains a large proportion of nitrogen and phosphoric acid, a possible explanation for its healing powers. Both substances can cause severe suppuration and cure it. Nitrogen is tissue-building in plants, whilst *Phosphoric acid* helps metabolism, needing acceleration in affected areas. After a cutting is made it is advisable to dip it in a *Calendula* solution to speed recovery and root growth. The moon calendar is invaluable help in determining the best time for striking from shoots and cuttings (see *Nitric acid* and *Phosphorus*).

Calendula in pest control has some properties worth considering: it repels asparagus beetle and does a lot of good in turf. Especially on bowling clubs' turf, with its unnatural environment, it discourages nematodes. The other varieties such as *Tagetus patula* and *Tagetes erecta* are highly regarded as natural nematicides. From the effects of "teas", like in biodynamic preparations, plenty of information has already been collated, to warrant the use of homoeopathic preparations.

APPEARANCE
Slightly or severely wilted after transplants.

WATER NEEDS
Low or normal, especially when striking cuttings.

In strikings or cuttings, *Calendula* will heal the wound and promote root growth. Calendula is part of the 'first aid' four-pack, a kit for plants containing *Arnica*, *Carbo vegetabilis*, *Silicea* and *Calendula*. These four remedies will cover most problems connected with transplants of plants.

RELATIONS
Compare: *Arnica*.
See also: *Nitricum acidum, Phosphorus.*

Camphora

Camphor. Cinnamonium camphora. Laurocerasus camphora. NO Lauraceae. Gum obtained from Laurus camphora. Solution in rectified spirit.

CLINICAL
Moths, wood worms, white ants, and other pests. Lodging, waterlogging, negative effects of cockroaches, ants.

GENERAL
Camphor is a white crystalline substance, which is harvested from the tree Laurocerasus camphora that grows in South-East Asia and Australia. There are some other odorous volatile products, found in different aromatic plants that have been given the same name. It is found either in longitudinal cavities in the heart of the tree or extracted from the leaves and twigs.

Grieve's herbal mentions that: "It is a well known preventive against moths and other insects, such as worms in wood; natural history cabinets are often made of it, the wood of the tree being occasionally imported to make cabinets for entomologists. (Grieve, 1931.)

As Camphor is a powerful remedy it should be used with caution because of the severe reactions it produces. It is often prescribed in the lower potencies, "but those whose knowledge of Camphor is confined to its coarser action will never understand what a great remedy it is when used according to its fine symptomatic indications and given in the higher potencies. " (Clarke, 1991.)

Because of its wide range of symptoms and the overlapping of primary and secondary reactions in humans, it is difficult to use there. In plants it produces enough symptoms to warrant its use in lodging, especially if caused by waterlogging, as Camphor is indicated for diseases arising from cold and damp weather.

The roots feel slimy, the slime being viscid, as is not found on healthy roots. The plant is excessively thirsty.

The capillary system does not work properly, thus interfering with transport of sugars to the roots and the uptake of nutrients into the plant. Consequently respiration and photosynthesis are defective and the plant slowly withers and collapses.

If the plant is its flowering stage, pollination occurs at night when pollen-feeding insects are at rest, thus interfering with fruit-setting.

Termites
Termites belong to the same family as cockroaches (not to the ants as their common name, the white ant, would suggest). They are related to the stonefly as well. They live in colonies which, contrary to all other colony dwellers such as ants and bees,

have not only a queen but also a king. The population is built up out of workers, soldiers and other castes. The soldiers have large heads and strong mandibles, but they are the ones that first scurry into safety when the nest is disturbed, especially so with the subterranean species.

Most species are 4 - 10 mm long, white or cream coloured and soft bodied. Depending on the species the nest is constructed either underground, in trees or in mounds. Most species can attack living or dead wood which is the reason why many wooden houses, or the stumps on which they are built, are a target for the termites.

Some species feed on fungi which they grow in underground tunnels, while still others chew on the roots of turf, field crops, and other vegetation. In spring they may swarm; males and females on the wing emerge in massive numbers from the nest, in a similar manner to ants. These mate, drop their wings, and setup a new nest as a royal couple. From the eggs the workers emerge which then build a new nest. In two to three years the egg-production speeds up with more egg-laying females Some queens become too large to move and only lay eggs. Some species manage up to 4000 eggs in twenty four hours.

In Australia they may attack a range of trees, mainly of the Eucalypt order. The reduction of native forests has brought them to human dwellings. *Camphora* is a good remedy against the termite. *Camphora* has been used on timber stock against termites with good results.

In the crude form it has been of service for hundreds of years. The camphor tree will remain free of termites, presumably because they do not like the smell. However, it is not only the smell that makes Camphor an excellent remedy against the termite. In the potencies it works just as well. In such fine dilutions there is no question of any smell, but it is possible that *Camphora* produces a repellent quality which is discernible to the termite. The insects are sensitive to the action of *Camphora*, with its prostration and debility - an unwanted phenomenon in a termite nest where there is constant work to do with the eggs, the larvae, the food reserves, etc. Here, a sleepy and debilitated state can be the death of the colony.

Cantharis

Spanish fly. NO Coleoptera. Trituration of live insect.

CLINICAL
Sunburn, blisters on leaves and petals. Fertiliser burns, water droplet burns, after bush fires, windburn. Bronze orange bug, rust chrysanthemum. Blister beetles on potatoes.

GENERAL
Cantharis upsets the generative sphere of the plant, causing burning. Consequently when the flowers appear burnt in hot weather, *Cantharis* is the remedy. It causes and cures an abundance of pollination from too long a stamen, readily absorbed by female flowers. Leaves and flower petals blister in the sun, especially after misting. Plant may have a burnt appearance. Fertiliser burns. After bush fires, to speed recovery and regrowth.

APPEARANCE
Burnt as after bushfire. Blisters on leaves and flower petals from fertiliser, water droplets or sunburn.

WATER NEEDS
High. Plant very thirsty. To replace sap lost in fires (*Carbo vegetabilis*).

FLOWERS AND FRUIT
Flowers abundant. As a reaction to fire, plant triggers off reproduction before it dies. Abundant pollen, good pollination. Fruits fail to mature, and drop before they set.

RELATIONS
Compare: *Bombyx*, *Carbo vegetabilis*.

Carbo Vegetabilis

Vegetable charcoal. Carbon (impure). Trituration.

CLINICAL
Slow recovery or dying plants after transplants. After severe mutilation through storm damage or mechanical injury. After rots. Decay, putrefaction, anthracnose. After loss of vital fluids. Nematodes.

GENERAL
Charcoal is, both in crude form and potencies, antiseptic and deodorant. The signs of decay and putrefaction are leading indications.

Carbo vegetabilis may also be much more than a rescuer of near-death plants. The carbon acts deeply on respiratory and chlorophyll cells, but except a stunted or wilted look due to capillary malfunction, does not exhibit noticeable symptoms elsewhere. Capillary collapse is an inevitable consequence of excessive carbon intake. (This finding is consistent throughout the carbons.)

Carbon forms the pivot of balance in relation to the other elements. It is not the resting point, but rather the rotating point - an axis - about which the shifting equilibrium of the other elements takes place. On the one hand the chemical uniformity of the carbon compounds presents a one sided and limited sphere of action, while on the other hand it presents an action upon all living entities. As such it is unlimited in its application.

All compounds, regardless the element of which it is formed, prove suitable to medicine. In plants this is of course restricted to those that play a role in plant life. Compounds usually act slower than pure elements, thus giving rise to a wider range of symptoms. Carbon exists in so many compounds that it can be considered the backbone in the treatment if plants and, possibly, in other living entities. Together with *Silicea* it forms a true agricultural polychrest. Carbon is the pillar of the entire organic world, while silica is the inorganic shell that encases the carbon. Carbon compounds are the most extensive in nature, not in the least because carbon can combine with itself.

The relation with silica is exquisite and extensive. Carbon is the building material and silica is the cement.

APPEARANCE
Wasted and wilted. Has nearly lost all leaves (not to be regarded in fall in deciduous trees), looks weak, burnt from bushfires, or dying from lack or excess of water. Desperate flowering (as in *Cantharis*) to reproduce before dying, yet too weak to produce fruit or seed. Fruits fall prematurely.

Streaks of reddish brown on the leaves, veins stand out; when a twig or leaf is broken, plant loses too much sap. *Carbo vegetabilis* was used extensively in Western Australia after transplants of blackboy trees and palms, with particularly good results on blackboy trees.

FLOWERS AND FRUIT
Desperate flowering. Long stamen, abundant pollen. Female flowers have impaired function. Premature falling of fruit, or no fruit development.

WATER NEEDS
In this instance, plants have to be considered individually as water needs may be low or high; especially in trees, each situation must be assessed by individual symptoms.

RELATIONS
Compare: *Arnica, Calendula*.
Complementary: *Silicea*

Chamomilla

German Chamomile. *Matricaria chamomilla*. NO Compositae. Tincture of whole plant.

CLINICAL
Damping off. Composting. Growth promoter. Contains a hormone that increases yeast. Wilting, wind rowing. Rusts, both yellow and red.

GENERAL
Grows besides roads and waste places on stony ground. "A painful increase in the sentient action followed by a considerable depression of the vital force. It increases the general sensitivity of the plant, a property that seems to give rise, secondarily, to various organic alterations that Chamomilla is capable of producing. "(Hahnemann, 1834.)

It is especially meant for plants that have been overdosed with pesticides. Debility is marked. The plant is hot and thirsty. The roots may be mouldy.

Damping off is the kind of debility that is typical of the *Chamomilla* state. It is often caused by an excess of nitrogen, which is usually given as a boost in the seedling stage. This causes a collapse of the seedlings, called 'damping off'. Plants treated with *Chamomilla* when very young become hardy against a number of plant diseases.

The roots may have a reddish appearance, be dry at the tip, or have froth on them. The plant is thirsty, the roots have a putrid smell. Sometimes there is a thick, yellowish mould, or blisters that break open. The plant appears to lack nutrients, yet application of fertiliser has little effect. The plant is wilted and very thirsty. Respiration impaired, oxygen release low. Contraction of respiratory problems. Photosynthesis impaired, starch and protein content low. Carbon binding deficient (*Calcarea carbonica, Magnesia carbonica, Kali carbonica, Ammonium carbonica*). Contraction of chlorophyll cells. From companion plant manuals and its use in the crude by Steiner, it can be inferred that the potencies should work even better.

Chamomilla has much in common with *Calcarea carbonica* because it covers acute stages of *Calcarea carbonica* problems, where calcium is deficient or in excess in the soil. It is the carbonate part that forms the link. It is thus equally a close relation with all carbonates including carbon itself. It is, in itself, hardly ever seen as a constitutional remedy but it has a wide range of action.

The farmer needs to give up NPK, use *Chamomilla* to enhance microbial life, and provide for distraction of pests. We recommend careful spraying, leaving weeds on the edges as an alternative food source for pests and an additional hiding place for pest predators. Reduction of food source always results in population decline.

Fungi must be given food lest they attack plants. A large proportion of fungi function to decompose debris, which is converted to nutrients for the crop. A thick layer of plant debris, such as straw, pea straw, bean straw, and compost can accomplish this.

MICROSCOPIC

There should be evidence of the above phenomena. Check carbon content and binding elements. (See also all other carbonates.)

NUTRITIONAL

Nutrient content low. Nutrients “locked up”, inability to assimilate. Food value is low due to low starch and protein content. Reduces the need for liming.

FRUITS AND FLOWERS

Flowering impaired, possible underdevelopment of ovaries, or insufficient production. Stamen is swollen, female flowers and parts do not function properly. Possibly deformed fruits which may rot on the tree due to over ripening.

WATER NEEDS

High.

RELATIONS

Compare: *Calcarea carbonica*.

Coccinella

Lady bird or lady beetle. Sunchafer. *Coccinella septempunctata*. NO Coleoptera. Tincture of the freshly crushed beetles.

CLINICAL
Aphids.

GENERAL
Aphids attack grains, fruits, vegetables and flowers.

Aphids are usually 1 - 2 mm long, although larger species also exist (4 - 5 mm). Different species have different colours - green, pink, deep yellow, grey or black. Some species have wings. Near the end of the body two tubes protrude, called cornicles, a feature particular to aphids. Aphids are viviparous (bearing live young) resulting in population explosions. When over-crowding occurs they develop wings to fly to other plants or other parts of the same plant.

Coccinella sprayed on the aphid rapidly diminishes the populations. Aphids pierce and suck, drawing sap from plants, preferably young shoots and buds, the latter producing deformed flowers. Some aphids form galls, attacking root system as well. Aphids are protected by ants and produce honey dew for them.

Population size depends on temperature and nutrient levels. At 15°C the females produce three young per day, increasing to six at 25°C. With high potassium and/or phosphorus this can increase to ten.

Coccinella has been used extensively with good results, usually requiring only a single dose. Overdosing will attract aphids to a plant with the result being repeated aphid infestations.

Coccus

Cochineal. *Coccus cacti.* NO Hemiptera. Trituration of the dried bodies of the female insect.

CLINICAL
All soft bodied scale.

GENERAL
Coccus, being a soft scale, is specific for treatment of soft scales. *Shellac* (a remedy I have made) is an example of a remedy for hard scales, as it is a product of a hard scale species. *Coccus* has been used on different species of scale living on different trees. Eucalypt scale (wattle tick, soft brown scale), scale on citrus trees, scale on bottle brush disappeared after a single dose. As with *Coccinella* care must be taken not to repeat the remedy.

There are some twenty types of soft scale, all of which can be treated with this remedy. It is the remaining hard scale (approximately ten species) that must be treated with *Shellac*. Thus, both *Coccus* and *Shellac* are somewhat generic.

Cochlearia

Horseradish. NO *Cruciferae*. Tincture of root.

CLINICAL
Brown rot on apples.

GENERAL
Only Rudolf Steiner has made anything resembling homoeopathic preparations for plants. He suggested about 50g of the crude substance diluted in 200l of water per hectare. From the homoeopathic way of potentising one can achieve a different level of refinement and fine tuned energy levels. Homoeopathy provides potencies that act more deeply, to give a more precise, more total cure.

Cochlearia armorica is beneficial to potatoes.

It is especially effective in persons who eat too much salt. In plants, this would indicate those over fed with too much salt, either as excessive fertilisers, or from salt water bores. Thus the leaves have excess water and salt, creating reduced photosynthesis and oxygen problems in respiration. The leaves distilled in water yield sulphurous essence. (See *Sulphur.*)

APPEARANCE
The roots have an offensive smell, have white moulds, and paralysis of function. Dry rots can appear anywhere, looks very sick. The plant absorbs readily any sodium, potassium and phosphorus, yet perspiration and evaporation are hardly possible. The leaves are bloated.

FRUITS AND FLOWERS
The flowers are stunted, both male and female parts are dysfunctional.

RELATIONS
Compare: *Sulphur.*

Coriandrum Sativum

Coriander. NO *Umbelliferae*. Tincture of fresh leaves and fruits.

CLINICAL
Aphids. It hinders the seed formation of fennel.

GENERAL
From Hylton's herbal it is noted that *Coriandrum Sativum* has a reputation of controlling aphids, while the plant itself seems immune to them. Together with Anise, which has the same reputation, they form a powerful duo that can be used either as a new remedy or as separate entities in the cure of the "aphid disease". As evident from *Phosphorus and Kali*, aphids attack plants that have an imbalance in either or both elements. Redressing that imbalance usually proves sufficient unless the plants are infested heavily. (Hylton, 1974.)

A lot of preparations attract both pest and diseases when conducting a proving on plants. A proving is the study of effects on plants, when they do not need a remedy. To conduct a proving, a plant is repeatedly sprayed with a homoeopathic remedy until the plants begin to show symptoms of either a disease, or a pest infestation. As the symptoms provoked are also those that can be addressed, we can in this way determine with great precision what pests and/or diseases the remedy is effective against.

Just as catch crops or lures can attract pests or disease from more valuable crops, a homoeopathic preparation can be sprayed on weeds to lure the pest or disease towards them. This aids both crop protection and weed eradication.

Weeds are seen as valuable allies in the natural setting, because pests and diseases can be directed towards them. Besides this, weeds fulfil other functions such as shelter for pest predators, green manure while decaying, and mulch and humus for the soil.

Weeds can indicate soil problems such as acidity, nutrient imbalance or toxicity. In general weeds act as restorers of the lost balance in excessive monocultures and, as such, are perfectly normal phenomena.

Bare soil cultivation is as unnatural as chemical farming. From the above it is clear that weeds are much more beneficial than is generally surmised, even in organic and biodynamic farming.

Cuprum Metallicum

Copper. Cu. Trituration. Elemental copper used for this preparation.

CLINICAL
Copper deficiencies and excesses. Fruit-drop, flower drop excessive. Only 1-2% of flowers have set fruit. Premature fruit-drop. Anomalies of flowering and fruiting. Early abscission of leaves.

GENERAL
Metallic copper works from within outwards. It ranks with the most important of those which relieve states arising from the 'striking inwards' of diseases. It is this power to relieve internal spasms which renders it appropriate in the state of collapse. *Cuprum* produces epidermic symptoms.

The plant seems to require more water and nutrients, there is chlorosis after excess iron, roots appear speckled white. Sometimes plants smell rotten although no rotting tissue can be found and no unusual symptoms are in evidence. Withertip can be seen as the state of cramp or spasm found in humans or animals. Affected shoots bend easily, wither and die. New shoots emerge lower in the tree or plant producing branches that look like mistletoe on the shoot tips. Because shoots do not mature, fruit setting and flowering are either totally absent or impaired. Fruit-drop in apples implicates fertilisers and copper deficiency, as well as hot dry summers, persistent wet, early winters, and competition between fruits. (Whitely, 1983.)

From agricultural publications it can be learned that copper deficiency and excess hinders the uptake of other nutrients, as long as the imbalance occurs in the plant. (Shorter and Cripps, 1985.)

Copper deficiency expresses itself as sterility of the pollen. It also increases the susceptibility to powdery mildew. Disease resistance depends on the age of the plant and the degree of the deficiency. (Bussler, 1981.)

Copper deficiency affects carbohydrate metabolism, nitrogen metabolism, cell-wall permeability and seed production. Young fruit trees are affected mainly on sandy soils. Speckling of the leaves. Withertip in grains; witch's broom appearance. Termination of all growth. Copper is antidoted by potassium.

Impaired photosynthesis, respiration and evaporation are some of the other problems associated with copper imbalance. Liming can be an aid in copper deficiency (see *Cup. sulph.*) Copper is an activator of some enzymes and may play a role in abscission, as some plant hormones and enzymes are triggered by copper.

In soil, copper becomes 'locked up' and unavailable to plants when nitrogen or ammonium are excessive.

The relations between copper and sulphur are expressed also through the sulphur based herbicides. It is generally accepted practise to use these in the beginning of the life cycle of a grain. Studies conducted in Western Australia (Robson and Snowball 1990, McCay and Robson 1992), and South Australia (Black and Wilhelm1991), showed that Sulfonylurea herbicides can reduce the uptake of copper and zinc in barley and wheat.

RELATIONS

Antidoted by: *Ammonium* preps, *Calcarea carbonica*, *Ferrum, Nitricum acidum, Phosphorus, Kali Nitricum,* and other *Kali* preps. *Sulphur.*

Inimical: *Molybdenum*, *Sulphur*, but not in *Cuprum sulphuricum*, *Zinc.*

Antidote to: *Ferrum, Phosphorus.*

Complementary: *Sulphur* but not in *Cuprum sulphuricum.*

Cuprum Sulphuricum

Sulphate of copper. $CuSO_4.5\ H_2O$. Trituration.

CLINICAL
Copper and Sulphur toxicity.

GENERAL
In his "Treatise on Dynamised Micro Immuno-therapy", O. A. Julian relates an experiment on plants performed by Prof. Netien of Lyon, and his assistant Mme Gravion, in 1965. They proved the activity of the infinitesimal doses of copper sulphate on plants intoxicated with the crude substance.

The dwarf beans were germinated in buckets filled with earth. Three times per week, a solution of unpotentised copper sulphate (20 mg/l) was watered in over a period of two months. The plants developed, flowered and bore fruit. Some of the treated beans were earmarked for experiment with homoeopathic dilutions receiving distilled water with either 5c, 7c, 9c, or 15c of *Cuprum sulphuricum* but, as a control, some of the seeds were treated with distilled water alone. Germination occurred normally for both treated and untreated plants.

After 3 days of observation, no difference was noted over all groups in regard to growth and development. The young plants were then placed in twice distilled water in culture phials, each plant in its own group. At the end of 3 more days, all treated groups were replaced in their corresponding homoeopathic solution.

On the eleventh day, photographic evidence was collected to verify that in comparison to the control, a very marked increase of development of the plants treated with homoeopathic dilutions of *Cuprum sulphuricum* had taken place. The increase was especially marked on the roots, whilst the difference between the potencies was much less than that between the treated and the control groups. Further evidence was collected on days 15 and 18. It has been shown that the homoeopathic dilutions of *Cuprum sulphuricum* have a positive action on the growth of bean seeds collected from plants intoxicated by crude copper sulphate.

The same experiment on seeds from "normal" plants gave much less convincing evidence. It can therefore be concluded that the diseased plants, with disturbed metabolism due to poisoning with copper sulphate, reveal the efficacy of homoeopathic treatment.

This research has been thoroughly verified on its merits by Netien, Gravion and Boiron, who have repeated the experiment using only the 14c potency of Cup. sulph.

Copper deficiency increases susceptibility to take-all (*Ophiobolus graminis*), when it is caused by excess of potassium. (Brennan, 1991, 1992.)

RELATIONS
Antidote to: *Ferrum, Phosphorus.*
Inimical: *Kali. Molybdenum, Zinc.*

Delia

Couchtip maggot. *Delia urbana*. NO Hymenopterae. Trituration of the live fly.

CLINICAL
Couchtip maggot fly.

GENERAL
Delia is an excellent remedy. It protects against this devastating pest on any lawn during the whole season with a single application.

APPEARANCE
Couchtip maggot. Eggs laid in the growing point of grass, hatch in spring and the larvae begin to eat the growing tip of the leaf. The result is bear patches and few runners with stunted look. The plant becomes straggly and weak. It can be easily pulled out and is often mistaken for a nutrient problem. The best visual sign consists of clouds of little black flies appearing above the lawn when it is walked upon.

WATER NEEDS
Before treatment little thirst because of short roots. After treatment give sufficient water to stimulate growth.

Equisetum

Horsetail. Scouring rush. *Equisetum hyemale*. NO *Equisetacae*. Trituration of whole plant. Trituration of ash. Tincture of whole plant chopped and pounded to pulp.

CLINICAL
Fungal diseases, mildews in grapevines, vegetables, roses and fruit trees. Pest and diseases in tomatoes. Leaf curl in peach.

GENERAL
Grows in wet, damp places, swamps, bogs, etc. Until now, the use of Equisetum has been restricted to the biodynamic preparations. It was decided to make this plant available in potency. To this end four tinctures were prepared.

Rudolf Steiner pointed out that burning the green plant in a quiet and steady flame produces ashes that contain up to 80% silica. This formed the mother tincture for the first preparation (*equisetum tosta*?) and potencies were made from this.

The whole plant was triturated for 20 hours with sugar of milk to make the second preparation at the 30x trituration. This served as mother tincture and further potencies were made of this.

Finally a tincture was made of the whole plant and potencies were made from this. It is evident that preparation 1 and 2 are more difficult to prepare than 3. They will show differences in their action as the burned substance is factually an oxide. Burning a substance causes oxidation, and the oxides in general have different properties to the pure element. (This can be shown by comparison of metals and their oxides.) The action of the oxide is very similar to that of *Silicea* (the main constituent).

From the biodynamic equisetum tea, we made a fourth potency range and the provings are consistent with Steiner's results with the crude form. The anti-fungal action is to be tested in a laboratory setting, and in the field. As results of this preparation come in, this materia medica will be extended.

Fungi in fruit trees must be sprayed after flowering. *Silicea* preparations will prevent fruit setting when applied too often and before flowering. As with all Silica preparations like *Polygonum*, use must be strictly accordance with instructions, and care must be taken to stick to the prescribed dosage in subsequent applications.

RELATIONS
See also *Silicea, Calcarea Silicea, Lapis albus, Silicic acid.*
Complementary: *Carbo vegetabilis.*

Ferrum

Iron. Fe. Trituration. Elemental iron used for this preparation. Trituration.

CLINICAL
Chlorosis. Pale, sickly plants that nearly fall over. Imperfect assimilation, impaired photosynthesis, protein content low. Fruit and vegetables have no taste. Bacterial blights, waterlogging, head-tipping, blasting, orange bug.

GENERAL
Iron is present in the blood and much of the food we eat daily. When *Ferrum* is given in potency to humans or animals, its first effect is to increase the amount of iron in the blood, stimulate the appetite, and augment body vigour. In green vegetables especially, it requires careful monitoring because this is another elementary remedy. Its secondary effects are opposite and give rise to its homoeopathic use.

Ferrum is needed for the process of photosynthesis. If there is an iron deficiency plants become chlorotic with a lack of chlorophyll. Iron is not a constituent of chlorophyll but is its catalyst. *Ferrum* inactivates *Calcarea* in favour of magnesium, which is an important constituent of chlorophyll.

As calcium represents Water, so iron represents Air, phosphorous is Fire, and silica and potassium are Earth. Chlorosis in plants, sterility, no fruit, no flowers, sickly stunted growth, pale, no strength to stand up, as in *Calcarea carbonica, Calcarea fluorata* and *Calcarea Phosphorus* with which it should be compared. Imperfect assimilation due to capillary problems, capillary collapse. Impaired photosynthesis due to absence of chlorophyll, consequently low protein content. This in turn leads to further weakening of the plants with inevitable collapse.

Iron is known as a nutritive remedy in some plant disorders, having an organopathic relationship to the capillary system. Digestive disorders with inability to assimilate calcium. It is not suited to all cases of chlorosis, or even the majority of them. It should, however, be given with discrimination and careful observation. Excess iron will cause anaemia and chlorosis and Ferrum preparations will severely aggravate in repeated doses.

It is suited to the type of chlorosis often seen in young plants with little capillary action. The appearance may be deceiving as the plant is healthy but with many pale leaves and a droopy appearance. There is paralysis of the capillaries which sets up a chlorotic weakness. Irritability of the tissues; they bruise easily. Plants are worse after watering and cold spells. In such cases the sulphide and phosphate are better than the pure metal unless it is very clearly indicated.

APPEARANCE

Pale sickly looking plants; no strength to stand upright. Chlorosis, low protein content, juvenile plants refuse to grow. Paleness of a dirty white or yellowish appearance.

CHEMICAL

Impaired photosynthesis, low protein content, systemic collapse of capillaries, paralysis of the capillary system. Impaired nutrition, little or no photosynthesis, low phosphorus and calcium content. Low sugar and starch.

FLOWERS AND FRUITS

Flowers have increased pollination yet are sterile. No fruits, or incomplete fruit setting. Immature fruit drops too early.

WATER NEEDS

Either want of water or worse for watering.

NOTE

Ferrum must be used with care. In general, *Ferrum phosphoricum* or *Ferrum sulphuricum* are better suited. *Ferrum* has some symptoms in common with *Calcarea, Silicea, Phosphorus, Kali* and *Ammonium* salts, *Manganese, Magnesium* and *Nitric acid*, because they form part of the properties of all living creatures, and as such, all of these remedies need careful study in their relationship to plants.

Ferrum preparations perform a similar function to the *Calcarea* group but are, however, very different and so cover a different range of diseases as well as cure some of the same diseases. Its relation to *Magnesia* is in a supportive role in photosynthesis. With *phosphorus* its relation is more in the same vein; oxidation.

RELATIONS

Antidote to: *Calcarea carbonica, Phosphorus.*
Inimical: *Kali, Phosphorus*, but not in *Ferrum phos.*
Antidoted by: *Cuprum, Manganum, Zinc.*
Complementary: *Magnesia.*
Compare: *Ammonium, Calcarea carbonica, Kali, Magnesia, Manganum, Nitricum acidum, Phosphorus.*

Ferrum Phosphoricum

Ferric phosphate. Ferrum phosphoricum album. Ferrous-ferric phosphate. White phosphate of iron (Schuessler's). Said to be a true ferric phosphate ($FePO_4$) as contrasted with the ordinary phosphate of iron which is a ferrous-hydric phosphate ($Fe(H_2PO_4)_2$). Trituration.

CLINICAL
For fresh wounds, contusions, sprains etc. For removal of excessive flow of sap, and vies with *Arnica* and *Calendula* as a first aid remedy. Indicated in the first stages of rust; reddish inflamed roots, dry under epidermis. Very thirsty plants that do not assimilate nutrients. Capillary congestion. Pale, straggly looking plants with many eruptions. Tan spot, blotches, bacterial blights, aphid, take-all.

GENERAL
This is Schuessler's preparation, used more often than ordinary phosphate of iron. Schuessler put *Ferrum phosphoricum* in the place of *Aconite, Belladonna, Gelsemium, Arnica* and others which correspond to circulation disorders.

Relaxation of tissue. It retains the features of other *Ferrum* preparations and caution is warranted.

Iron and its salts possess the property of attracting oxygen. The iron in the sap takes up produced oxygen which it transports at night to be exhaled by the plant. During the day a plant takes up carbon dioxide from the air. The sulphur contained in the sap and capillaries assists in transferring oxygen from all the cells containing iron and sulphate of potassium. When the molecules of iron contained in the cells of the cambium have suffered a disturbance through some injury or wound, the affected cells grow flaccid. If this affection takes place in the annular fibres of the capillaries, they are dilated and sap is increased. When cells are brought back to normal with *Ferrum phosphoricum* the cells can cast off disease. When the flaccid cells in the cambium receive *Ferrum phosphoricum* the normal tension in the capillaries is restored. The swollen vessels are reduced to their normal size and thus the spots and blotches disappear leaving only a little scar tissue as shown from clinical tests.

APPEARANCE
As other spots and blotches have already been covered, only bacterial blights will be discussed in this section.

Bacterial blights. Halo spot (Pseudomonas spp.).
Small green oval water-soaked spots on the leaves and sheaths up to 10 mm across. The centres of the spots change to straw or brown colour. A small green water-soaked halo appears on the surrounding leaf. Later the patches become more brown and join together in irregular patterns.

Stripe-blight. (Xanthomonas translucens)
Similar to halo spot but elongated without halo. First water-soaked, and then brown stripes with yellow margins which later join in irregular patterns. Emerged florets appear mottled, brown or white (*Aconite, Belladonna*) and may be sterile. Leaves wither and die.

Blight bacteria survive on seed and debris. They spread by rain splash or leaf contact. Aphids can also act as carriers. Moist weather favours development and spread. Dry weather stops spread.

WATER NEEDS
It is advisable not to water much in dry weather to stop spread. The plant is very thirsty and wilts. Use trickle system.

FLOWERS AND FRUITS
Either abundant pollen or complete absence. Premature flowering, difficult flowering, difficult setting of the fruit.

RELATIONS
It is not only *Ferrum* preparations that are indicated in such diseases, the *Ferrum phosphoricum* debilitation and suppurative processes paint a perfect picture of the capabilities of Phosphorus to upset the epidermis with blackish ulcers. *Nitric acid* and *Kali carbonica*, *Natrum sulphate*, and *Natrum carbonica* can be indicated for similar symptoms. Although normally *Phosphorus* is the antidote of *Ferrum*, here it is seen as a complement because the normally antagonistic actions are here combined. This creates a substance which not only acts on the capillaries - hence the rots - but is also a stimulant for flowering and fruit setting.

Ferrum Sulphuricum

Sulphate of iron. $FeSO_4$. Trituration of freshly prepared crystals or solution.

CLINICAL
Impaired photosynthesis, deformed flowers, straggly, twisted, deformed appearance. Tree cancer. Tree-hoppers, moulds and mildews, black point, septoria blotch, aphids, scale, mites, bud worm, citrus mite, elephant weevil.

GENERAL
Ferrum sulphuricum corresponds, like *Calcarea carbonica*, *Calcarea fluorica* and *Silicea fluorica*, to the condition of cancer in trees. Nutrients are not taken up. It may be suited to removing mercury from plants or modifying mercury uptake in plants. All symptoms are worse in summer, on warm days, at night and in the morning. Afternoons generally give the best appearance. The roots may appear discoloured, red, or have bright red papular eruptions. Swelling of parts of the roots. There is a dry feeling under the epidermis of the root. (In healthy plants, this is moist.) Nutrient uptake is impaired or absent. Moulds of all kinds; powdery mildews, downy mildew, grey mould of all species, sooty mould of all species, some black moulds. The exception here is slimy moulds which, on account of similarity in appearance, have been grouped with snails and slugs and covered by *Helix tosta*.

APPEARANCE
Grey mould (Botrytis spp.). This fungus produces sclerotia and can be present throughout the whole year in plant debris. Grey furry surface indicates spore formation. Cool, humid conditions are required. The spores are spread by wind. All above ground parts are affected although there is an affinity for fruit. Pears develop a soft brown rot and the spores develop typically grey and powdery, assuming conditions are favourable.

Dying flowers are often the first affected and form the centre from whence the fungus spreads. In cyclamen, attack usually begins at soil level because of the higher humidity. On lily leaves, oval or round spots, yellowish or reddish brown, and visible on both the top and bottom of the leaves. In damp conditions, the colour fades with an increase in size. Gradually, the spots converge and the leaf dies. Stems can be spotted and break when they converge. Affected buds produce distorted flowers that wither and drop; many of them brown or destroyed. In humid conditions spores will be formed.

Powdery mildew (*Alternaria* spp.), sooty mould-black point (Bipolaris spp.) fungi:
The embryo end of the growth darkens. It is caused by the two fungi and lives on decaying grasses and is very common. Spores are carried everywhere. Rain during grain development and filling enables the fungus to infect the seed or grain, and develops slowly during the ripening process. The grains may still be used for seed stock because 'the germination is rarely affected'. (Grains R&D Corp. 1992.)

However, this makes the grain more susceptible and a larger amount of grain can be affected. Continued use of this infected seed will result in sterility and crop loss. It is better, when using infected seed, to spray with *Ferrum phosphate* shortly after seeding to reduce infection and thus have clean seed for the next crop. In this way resistance is built up and carried into the next generation, thus making susceptibility obsolete. What takes enormous amounts of time and money, through genetic engineering, can be achieved cheaply and quickly through homoeopathic treatment.

Septoria blotch (*Mycosphaerella* spp., NO Fungi). Blotches on leaves, irregular in shape, tan to brown, occasionally silvery with yellow rims. Along leaf veins blotches have straight margins. Black specks, which are fruiting bodies, can be seen inside the blotches. The fungus survives in wheat residues. After rain in autumn, the spores are produced in great quantity, spread by wind, and can be carried over long distances in waterlogged areas, particularly in the hills where spores are carried by running water. Infection is most likely in newly sown crops. After three weeks to a month, small black fruiting bodies form on the leaves. This is the time to spray *Ferrum sulphuricum*. In moist conditions spores are produced and are carried from leaf to leaf by rain splash. In heavy rainfall crop loss of up to 30% has been recorded. It is much less likely to spread in dry spells lasting for up to a month. It does not affect grazing animals since it is a less lethal fungus than Secale or Ustilago. It is more similar to black spot than to ergot or smuts.

Glume blotch, septoria nodorum blotch (*Leptosphaeria nodorum*):
Blotches on leaves that are yellow or tan to brown, oval shaped, turning to grey as they enlarge. Leaves die with yellow tops. Chlorotic appearance. Fruiting bodies are grey-brown with specks within blotches. Later in the season the stems and glumes become infected. Heavy infection often results in loss of the whole ear. Grey and brown blotches with shrivelling of the grain. Seed loss may be complete. Fruiting bodies with spores are frequently found on both stem nodes and glumes.

The fungus survives in stubble and stalk debris. It affects wheat, barley, barley-grass and brome grass. Spores develop after rain and are wind dispersed over large areas. Early sown crops are easily infected. The ideal environment for infection is during warm, wet weather with heavy frequent rain. Spores spread from plant to plant by rain splash.

RELATIONS
Compare: *Sulphur*.
Antidote to: *Calcarea, Cuprum, Phosphorus*.
Inimical: Kali, *Molybdenum, Phosphorus*.
Antidoted by: *Cuprum, Manganum, Zinc*.

Helix Tosta

Toasted snail. NO *Helicidae*. Trituration.

CLINICAL
Snails and slugs and slimy moulds.

GENERAL
Snails are reported to have traditional virtue in curing consumption. Homoeopaths have put the remedy to the test by potentising it. Plants, when consumed by snails and slugs, present a perfect picture of respiratory deficiency. This remedy has had extensive clinical verification in the field. It was found to protect plants from snail attack when watered in or sprayed, so that the plant takes up the remedy.

Helix tosta 6x protects plants to the degree that snails will pass previously sprayed plants to eat only untreated plants. No other preparation works four months after one single dose, even in heavy rain. *Helix tosta* was tested extensively at herb farms and back yard gardens. When sprayed on the plant infested with snails, it destroys the shell making it soft and slimy. On account of similarity and appearance, slimy moulds should also come under its action, but this has not yet been verified.

Helix tosta does not affect the small native snail, but only the so called Italian snail and the slug.

Hyssop

Hyssopus officinalis. NO Labiatae. Tincture of the whole plant.

CLINICAL
Bacterial rots, blights, cabbage butterfly trap, general insect repellent. Respiratory problems. Best action in viticulture.

GENERAL
Originally a native of the hilly regions of Italy, hyssop is a good companion plant for grape vines, increasing their yield. Steiner uses a tea on bacterial diseases. In potency it should prove to have a wide ranging action considering its variety of uses in crude form. Hyssop and radish are incompatible. Blue hyssop is the best insect repellent, followed by pink and white. This information is found in companion plant manuals and the potencies should confirm it. (Philbrick and Gregg, 1966.)

On account of its herbal properties it is also effective in respiratory ailments.

Kali Carbonicum

Potassium carbonate. K_2CO_3. Solution. Trituration.

CLINICAL
Fibrous tissue is weak; flowering and fruit setting impaired. Capillary engorgement, chlorosis, worse in acidic soils. Bronze orange bug.

GENERAL
The potassium salts form a large part of a plant's diet, and is therefore a remedy of prime importance where nutrition is impaired or imbalanced. Although differences will be found in its respective constituents, as is the case with the *Calcarea* and *Ferrum* preparations, yet the *Kali* symptoms run throughout the pathogenesis. (See also *Cham.*)

Caution is recommended with all tissue salts, as indiscriminate use leads to disaster. Witness the excess application of NPK which has produced much disease on plants and consequently animals and man. In potassium excess and deficiencies alike, *Kali carbonica* works well, but is dependent on the plant species concerned.

It is better to use the old fashioned open-pollinated varieties to maintain a healthy seed stock. Hybrids become more prone to disease through inbreeding and this results in quality loss. Resistant varieties of cereals are only resistant against one or two diseases and only for a few years.

Potassium was seen in Europe (Denmark) to increase ear-number, but reduce grain weight in higher than normal applications. Drought combined with excess potassium during ripening reduces yield. Both grain weight and number per ear was negatively affected. It stimulates leaf growth, thus increasing dry matter. (Anderson et al. 1992)

Cotton varieties which fruit faster and have higher yields, develop potassium deficiencies even with extra applications. The cotton bolls will then withdraw potassium from the leaves, leading to their breakdown as well as a reduction in the quality and quantity of cotton per plant. (Hake, 1991.)

Potassium carbonate, sometimes called 'vegetable alkali', exists in all plants, and was originally obtained from the ashes after burning wood. The potassium salts have more specific relation to the solid tissues than to the fluids in the plant. Both excess and deficiency can cause the following symptoms which correlate with the findings of Mason and Gartrell. (Undated publication, Department of Agriculture, WA.)

The fibrous tissue is especially affected. It corresponds to conditions in which these tissues are relaxed. It affects flowering and fruit setting, the capillary system, leaves, stems, twigs, branches and roots. It is indicated in situations where plants seem to "give out". Chlorosis is an important feature. The plant is worse in windy or cold weather. Problems alternate, weak plants with epidermis watery and very pale. Plants seem better during the day and may wilt at night. Vesicles on the roots. Acidic soils exacerbate the problem.

In potassium deficiency there is a sudden collapse of the top layer of cells on the older leaves. There are waterlogged blotches which turn into dead patches. Chlorosis extending from the margin inwards. The leaves and later the flowers wither and die. Total capillary collapse. Also puckering of the older leaves: wilting leaves have a dull sheen. (Mason and Gartrell, undated.)

Grass tetany is caused by anomalies in the ratio potassium:[calcium and magnesium]. This discrepancy serves as a guide to potentially lethal pastures. It was found that when this ratio exceeds 1:1 in grasses, cattle death ensues. Different plant species as well as different soils give different critical K:(Ca + Mg) values. (Lewis and Sparrow, 1991.)

FLOWERS AND FRUITS

Flowers are either abundant in pollen, or have none at all. Fruits drop prematurely, fail to set or ripen. Leaves have a dry epidermis, feel brittle, and have yellow or red spots, which are corrosive and destroy surrounding tissue.

Kali carbonica is indicated in any plants that either lack or have too much potassium and calcium. In calcium rich soils, where potassium gets "locked up", in soils with poor calcium content, nutrients do not assimilate. Many nutrient problems,

Kali carbonica is associated with many diseases, deficiencies and when soil is poor. Again, caution is important when using any Kali preparation.

RELATIONS

Antidote to: *Boron, Borax.*

Antidoted by: *Calcarea carbonica* and other *Calcarea* and *Natrum* preps.

Inimical: *Boron, Borax., Calcarea carbonica, Calcarea Phosphorus, Calcarea Silicate, Calcarea sulphate, Ferrum, Manganum, Natrums.*

Kali Muriaticum

Chloride of potassium. KCl. Trituration solution.

CLINICAL
Grey moulds, powdery mildew, downy mildew.

GENERAL
Schuessler (1984), says of the salt: "It is contained in nearly all cells and is chemically related to fibrin. It will dissolve white or greyish white secretions of the mucous membrane. When the cells of the epidermis lose molecules of potassium chloride in consequence of a morbid irritation, then the fibrin comes to the surface as a whitish grey mass; when dried this forms a mealy covering. If irritation has seized upon the tissues under the epidermis, then fibrin and serum are exuded causing the affected spot on the epidermis to rise in blisters. Similar processes will take place in and below the epithelial cells." (Schuessler, 1984.)

Kali muriaticum manifests its action in about equal proportion of its constituents. The keynote is whiteness of secretions, exudations and eruptions of the tissues. The next important keynote is toughness; mildews are tough and threadlike.

As *Kali muriaticum* is one of the main constituents of NPK, providing the potassium to the soil, it is evident that this remedy is of prime importance in the removal of problems originating from excess potassium. Potassium excess can block a plant's uptake of magnesium, because the potassium binds to it and it becomes unavailable.

Because *Kali muriaticum* is a chloride, a salt, it is implicated in salination problems. Salination is a problem in itself, where the usual mix of salts makes treatment rather problematic. Chloride and sodium bind easily, and *Kali* is depicted as the remedy with the largest amount of connections with the largest group of elements, salts and acids, to further complicate the picture. What is found in different salt lakes and salt pans created by poor agricultural methods, land clearing and the rise of the water table is another complicated environmental problem, which needs careful study and assessment.

As with the nitrogen and phosphorus portions of NPK, *Kali* is implicated in the occurrence of pests. The phosphate content in NPK is the most strongly indicated in pest attacks, leading to a study of the differences in plants fed NPK, if *Kali muriaticum* was given. Thus manganese and potassium levels were tested and susceptibility to pests and diseases was investigated.

Moulds and mildews being the most salient features so far, we have included these in the pathogenesis. Potassium is antagonistic to boron, thus reducing the boron uptake and causing crown rot in turnips, and sickle leaf and hollow stem in cauliflower. Potassium and magnesium are mutually antagonistic; too much of either reduces the uptake of the other. Although their actions as such do not show any relation in the materia medica, it might prove very helpful to follow up on soil analysis with the addition of an element that, homoeopathically, will trigger the uptake. It is useless to apply high NPK and then follow with boron or magnesium; it will only add to the soils' woes, as this type of practise is the only solution open to the farmer.

A homoeopathic remedy will act on both plants and soil microbiology, because a microbe induced into inactivity by NPK will be activated by the homoeopathic dynamis. In plants it will be visible in the restoration of health which is only possible if the deficient element has been taken up. Therefore, the restoration of health in the plant automatically includes the diseases of soil microbial life as they are interdependent.

Symptoms of potassium deficiency include sudden or delayed collapse of the top layer of cells in older leaves with waterlogged areas, which later become dead patches. These leaves then become pale and turn yellow at the leaf margins extending towards the centre. The areas around the mid rib and veins remain green the longest. The older leaves begin to die, followed by the younger ones. Flower heads wither and die till the whole plant is affected and dies. Some plants are more susceptible than others, even different species within the same family.

APPEARANCE
Greyish white moulds on roots, stems or leaves. Plants affected by mildew, roots may be affected too. Swollen capillary system. Dry flour-like moulds and mildews. Burns of all degrees.

FLOWERS AND FRUITS
Flowers mouldy, fruits with mildews.

WATER NEEDS
Normal.

The Kali salts are the most extensively dealt with in homoeopathy. This great variety shows us that potassium may lock up many more salts not known to affect plants, and the relationship they form with other elements may lead us to new discoveries in plant chemistry and biology. Although we may not understand these relationships fully as yet, it will certainly help if more research is directed at their unravelling. In plants different relationships exist as in humans.

The difficulty is that it is not necessarily a wise decision to completely discard all the relationships as we know them. After all, an antidote is always the antidote, because it is the remedy that is antidoted, or so we assume - basically from the instructions of Hahnemann in regards to the manufacture of different remedies. At the same time it can also be assumed that we antidote the action of the remedy in the body, in which case we have a different situation in plants, where what is normally an antidote or an inimical, we now see as complementary.

The particular situation will reveal to us, in what way that situation has to be assessed. This means that also here - i.e. in plants - it is the patient and not the disease which needs assessment and treatment. Individualisation is one of the laws of homoeopathy which does not change when treating other living entities.

Natrum and *Kali* are normally inimical, while *Natrum* is also the antidote to *Kali*.

RELATIONS
Compare: *Natrum muriaticum.*
Antidote to: *Magnesia.*
Antidoted by: *Ferrum, Manganum, Natrum muriaticum.*
Inimical: *Natrum muriaticum.*

Kali Nitricum

Saltpetre. Nitrate of potassium. KNO_3. Trituration or solution.

CLINICAL
Nitrogenous soils, excess nitrogen and related problems. Excess potassium. Yellowing from nitrogen deficiency.

GENERAL
Many plant diseases are caused by excess nitrogen such as eyespot, powdery mildew. It causes irregularities in flowering and fruit setting, photosynthesis irregularities, and fluid uptake difficulties. The roots may show mouldy patches. Plants are thirsty and wilt easily when fluids are used up during droughts.

This remedy can do much to balance the nutrients, lower the nitrogen content in the plant, aid photosynthesis, and enhance the protein content. The excess pollination will be regulated and fruits will set and ripen properly.

Kali nitricum can be helpful in sulphur deficiency when nitrogen is excessive in the plant. This is only possible when there is also a potassium imbalance. (Bussler, 1964.)

RELATIONS
Compare: *Nitric acid* and *Ammonium* preparations.
Complementary: *Sulphur.*

Kali Permanganicum

Potassium Permanganate. $KMnO_4$. Solution. Trituration.

CLINICAL
Excessive wilting, with no improvement from watering. Pale striping from manganese deficiency. Grey speck. Apple leaf hopper. Aphids. Blister mite. Two-spotted mite. Mildews. Slugs, snails.

GENERAL
This is another potassium salt which is an oxidising agent and which assists in photosynthesis and protein enhancement. The roots appear too dry under the epidermis. The plant is thirsty as one would expect from the wilted appearance, yet watering does not seem to help. It has a similar action as iron (see *Ferrum* preparations). It has a marked power over oxidation. (Leeser, 1932.)

The normal relation of *Manganum* being the antidote to *Kali*, is here totally suspended. Rather they have here assumed the role of complements, as the oxidising property is not the antagonistic agent which it is in the normal functioning of potassium. As a plant food, potassium is here relegated to a secondary role. The manganese component takes on the lead role in remediating the lack of oxidation which manifest in the development of mildews and grey speck. Lack of oxidation brings on the pests; they thrive on plants that have the type of wilting seen here. A plant lacking oxygen is as good as food for pests because it has no resistance. The taking up of oxygen enables the plant to process its food, while a lack brings on "constipation" or "diarrhoea". This means that its carbohydrates are either unavailable - the plant cannot transport them from the roots to where they are needed - or are processed too fast.

RELATIONS
Compare: *Manganum.*
Inimical: *Ferrum, Natrum muriaticum*; but not *Manganum.*
Antidoted by: *Natrum muriaticum.*

Kali Phosphoricum

Phosphate of potassium. K_2HPO_4. Trituration. Solution.

CLINICAL
Chlorosis. Photosynthesis impaired. Potato gangrene. Bloated leaves full of fluid. Purpling of leaves in Phosphorus deficiency. Environmental stress.

GENERAL
Schuessler tells us that *Kali phosphoricum* produces irregularities in the capillary system. Nutritional problems; nutrients are not taken up the plant is weak gangrenous, and straggly. The immunity of the plant is greatly impaired; drought, stress, frost and temperature shock affect the plant profoundly. Head tipping, sterility from blasting, and waterlogging are some of the environmental stress symptoms associated with *Kali phosphoricum* imbalance. The generative sphere is strongly affected, flowers pollinate excessively or not at all whilst fruit setting is slow or only partial. Purpling in barley due to phosphorus imbalance. This last is also the cause for susceptibility to environmental stress and flowering and fruiting irregularities. The capillary problems were positively affected in field tests.

RELATIONS
Compare: *Ammonium Phosphoricum, Calcarea Phosphoricum, Chamomilla, Ferrum Phosphoricum, Magnesia Phosphoricum, Phosphorus*.
Antidoted by: *Ferrum, Manganum, Natrum muriaticum.*
Inimical: *Ferrum, Manganum, Natrums.*

Kali Sulphuricum

Potassium sulphate. K_2SO_4. Trituration.

CLINICAL
Impaired photosynthesis. Rust and its results. Chlorosis. Beginning stages of ergot. Banana rust thrips.

GENERAL
Kali sulphuricum acts reciprocally with iron in the transfer of exhaled oxygen, and is contained in all cells containing iron. A deficiency of *Kali sulphuricum* results in desquamation of the cells of the epidermis and epithelium which have been loosened because of excess oxygen remaining during the day. After rust. When a sulphate and any oxide of iron come in contact with decomposing organic matter, they surrender their oxygen and form a sulphate of iron. After more oxidation this further decomposes into sulphuric acid and a single oxide of iron. The plants suffer most on hot days and during summer. From the pathogenesis, this remedy may be effective in the first stages of ergot disease when the sticky, shiny droplets are produced during flowering.

APPEARANCE
Rust or chlorosis, first stages of ergot disease.

WATER NEEDS
Normal.

FLOWERS AND FRUITS
In ergot when the sugary, shiny droplets are formed during flowering.

RELATIONS
Compare: *Ferrum* preps.
Complementary: *Ferrum* preps.
Antidoted by: *Natrums*.
Inimical: *Ferrum, Manganum, Natrums*.

Lactic Acid

Milk acid. Lacticum acidum. $HC_3H_5O_3$. Dilution.

CLINICAL
Mosaic virus and mildews. Red spider mite.

GENERAL
Lactic acid, 'was discovered by Scheele in sour milk, the result of spontaneous fermentation of sugar of milk under the influence of casein. It is also met with in many vegetable products which have turned sour.' (Hering, 1991.)

Lactic acid is a bactericide of the first order, particularly in plants. If *lactic acid* slightly oxidises it produces pyruvic acid which functions as the trigger for the Krebs cycle in plants. *Lactic acid* in potencies should, for that reason, play an important role in the respiration of plants. Pyruvic acid plays an important role in the chemistry of biological processes. It is an intermediate in the conversion of proteins, carbohydrates and fats. It is found in abundance in cucumbers.

Mosaic virus can be kept under control through the use of milk sprays (Conacher, 1991). Conacher recommends 1 part of milk and 9 parts of water, in repeated applications, ten days apart.

To control mildew, 1 part of milk and 2 parts of water are used. To cover $20m^2$ it is advised to use 0.5l of milk in 1l of water. Therefore a hectare ($10,000m^2$) requires 250l of milk, which would be cost prohibitive. Potencies of *lactic acid* will act equally well at a fraction of the cost.

Red spider mite can be treated with *Bovista* or *Tromb*.

RELATIONS
Compare *Salicylic acid.*
Complementary: *Acetic acid, Oxalic acid.*

Lapis Albus

Silicofluoride of calcium. $CaSiF_6$. Taken from Lapis Albus (a species of gneiss found by Grauvogl in the mineral springs of Gastein and named by him. The waters flow over the gneiss formations into the valley of Aachen where goitre and cretinism abound). Trituration.

CLINICAL
Cancer in trees. Scarring on bark, tumors on roots, potato rot. Black leg potato, black bulb rot, black rot, radish black rot, black spot roses, strawberry blossom-end rot, potato gangrene. Rots and decaying diseases in all species. Some forms of mosaic virus. All rots are dry rots.

GENERAL
The salient features of *Lapis* belong to rots and the generative organs, the flowers being absent, stunted, shrivelled, and otherwise deformed, if the plant gets to that stage. Any soil, in which your plant gets sick should lie fallow for one year, and be provided with humus or humus forming aids. Rots of nearly all kinds, cancers on trees with no ulceration, mottled and rotten leaves. Scarring of bark, pale appearance.

APPEARANCE
As all dry rots are similar, only three examples will be given as symptoms are identical for any part of the plant.

Bitter rot apple (Glomerella cingulata): Signs of disease come on late, near ripening. They consist of small brown spots spreading rapidly to cover one third of the fruit in two to three days. In humid conditions this results in the growth of masses of pink spores which form concentric circles. It can completely dry out the fruit as the skin sinks in deeper and deeper, till the mummification is complete with the fungus surviving in a self-made cocoon till next season. When the temperature drops below 20^0C and after sufficient rain, the cocoon collapses and the spores are blown out by the wind and back onto the trees. Willy Sharp, Gravenstein and Granny Smith are mostly affected, but other apples can as easily be affected.

Black root, radish (Aphanomyces raphani): This fungus produces irregular black patches on the root. These areas may become sunken. Sometimes the root may split although the tissue remains firm. Warm, moist conditions are most favourable for this disease. The fungus can survive several years in the soil, and is spread by rain splash and running water. Penroot radish is more often attacked than bulb root.

Blossom-end rot, tomato: The symptoms only occur on the blossom end of the fruit. The area becomes brown, tough and sunken. Sometimes, as in egg tomatoes, the effect is entirely internal and shows only a dark brown interior through the skin. It occurs halfway through the maturation process.

These symptoms indicate that there is a lack of calcium; the fruit cannot form. The calcium content in the soil may be too low, the soil too acidic, or the levels of NPK are too high. There may be a fluctuating water supply, or too many leaves forming simultaneously with fruit (available calcium goes to the leaves). *Lapis* will redress the uptake of calcium where sufficient levels are present. The pH has little to do with the health of a plant as at biodynamic farms healthy plants have grown in a pH of 3. 5. *Lapis*, containing calcium silicofluoride, stops the dry suppuration and balances calcium uptake, or, alternatively, if not available in abundance, regulates the plant's use of it.

It is the dry rots and tree cancers that *Lapis* will do much to redress. At the first sign of infected tomatoes, immediately spray *Lapis* 6x and it will be nipped in the bud.

As with *Calcarea* preparations, *Lapis* should be used with the utmost caution. It cannot be stressed enough that very small doses exert a great influence over plants, particularly the tissue salts, because they form essential building blocks of the plant.

RELATIONS
Compare: *Ammonium carbonica, Calcarea carbonica, Chamomilla, Kali carbonica, Magnesia carbonica, Natrum carbonica*.
Antidoted by: *Ammonium* preps. *Nitricum acidum, Sulphur*.
Complementary: *Silicea, Natrum silicofluoricum*.
Antidote to: *Ferrum, Magnesia, Manganum, Zinc*.
Inimical: *Magnesia, Phosphorus*.

Magnesia Carbonica

Carbonate of magnesium. $MgCO_3$. Trituration.

CLINICAL
Wilting, temperature shock, frost shock. Chlorosis, dirty yellow. Windburn, damping off.

GENERAL
Magnesia carbonica is sensitive to environmental stress, as in temperature shock, like *Kali phosphorica.* The main difference between the two is that *Magnesia carbonica* is much more sensitive to environmental stress. Puny, sickly looking plants which do not thrive on acidic soils or have been given unsuitable nutrients. Nitrogen given in seedling stage leads to collapse. There are vesicles on the roots, which are too dry under the epidermis. The plants are very thirsty and wilt more in the evening when the sun sets. The flowers have incomplete or no stamen, causing impaired or absent fruiting. Photosynthesis is impaired, protein content is low. Capillary system is engorged, its action impaired.

Magnesia is inimical to *Natrum muriaticum* and *Kali* and an excess of either causes magnesium deficiency or, vice versa, causes a reduction in the uptake of sodium in the coastal areas where salt water bores cause problems with salination. Liming may also cause Magnesia deficiencies, especially when it is excessive. Delbet considers Magnesium to be important in germination. Magnesium is abundant in the seeds of plants while the corm contains more than the straw. (Delbet, 1956.)

Virus infections can severely affect plant nutrition levels. Nitrogen, phosphorus, magnesium and zinc concentrations usually increase while potassium levels decrease. (Kaplan and Bergman, 1985. Shattuck, 1987.)

Magnesium stands between the *Kali* and *Calcarea* preparations, partaking in its action to *Kali* when found in association with it, or alternatively partaking to calcium if it is found to associate there. Leeser considers magnesium to be of physiological significance most strongly in plants. In organic form it is found in the chlorophyll. It plays a role in the assimilation of CO_2 in the oxidation of the carbon compounds. It is inimical to sodium and potassium. (Leeser, 1936.)

The symptoms of magnesium deficiency appear rapidly. (cf *Aconite* and *Bell.*) Yellowing of the leaves, marbling between the veins. These spots become necrotic. The appearance is similar to yellow dwarf virus symptoms. The oldest leaves are least affected, later also the younger leaves. The veins and the mid rib remain green. The leaves fold backward as they die. At the back of the leaves the interveinal areas are pink. (Mason and Gartrell, undated.)

Magnesium is more a food nutrient than a trace-element, for it is needed in quantity. NPK and magnesium are, as such, closely related, much as the micro-nutrients.

Deficiency shows as yellowing of the leaf tips and margin, leaving a dark green tongue at the leaf base. Chlorosis increases and leaf scorch sets in on the margin. Older leaves are most affected. This problem is prominent in apples: Lady Williams, Yates, Red and Gold Delicious, Jonathan and Abas. (Mason and Gartrell, undated.)

RELATIONS

Compare: *Aconite, Ammonium muriaticum, Belladonna, Ferrum muriaticum, Kali muriaticum, Natrum muriaticum.*

Inimical: *Calcarea carbonica, Kali carbonica, Kali muriaticum, Kali Phosphorica, Kali sulphuricum, Natrum carbonica, Natrum muriaticum, Phosphorus.*

Complementary: *Calcarea carbonica, Kali* preps, *Nitricum acidum, Phosphorus, Zinc.*

Antidoted by: *Manganum.*

Magnesia Muriatica

Chloride of magnesium. $MgCl_2$. Solution. Trituration.

CLINICAL
Salination problems. Puny, rickety plants, chlorosis.

GENERAL
Magnesia muriatica has many features in common with *Natrum muriaticum*, and sea water. It has a very bitter taste. The roots of the plant appear swollen and are dry under the epidermis. The plant needs frequent watering. Photosynthesis is impaired, and leaves may show signs of rust.

The flowers may not develop fully or have distorted stamens, whilst fruit setting is greatly impaired.

RELATIONS
Compare: *Natrum muriaticum, Kali. muriaticum.*
Inimical: *Calcarea carbonica, Kali. muriaticum, Natrums, Phosphorus.*
Antidoted by: *Manganum.*
Complementary: *Calcarea carbonica, Kali* salts.

Magnesia Phosphorica

Phosphate of magnesium. $Mg_3(PO_4)_2$. Trituration. Solution.

CLINICAL
Chlorosis, yellowing, bronzing and shedding of the leaves. Mites.

GENERAL
Magnesia phosphorica, according to Schuessler and by analogy in plants, is contained in the sap, the structural tissues and chlorophyll. Disturbance in the molecular structure results in paralysis of the capillaries. Because excess potassium will lock it into the soil, a lack of magnesium phosphate will result in disturbances of metabolism, evaporation, and photosynthesis. It has a strong family resemblance to *Magnesia carbonica* and *Magnesia muriaticum*. The plants suffer most in cold rainy weather, from waterlogging. Cankers of the roots, with cracked epidermis. The plant seems to wilt or cannot hold itself upright. Vitality is greatly depressed.

From research it has become evident that phosphorus cannot be taken up without magnesium, nor can it be properly distributed. It is the second main article in the diet of man and animal, whilst it holds the approximate fifth place in plants. Without it no living entity can live properly and they appear “clapped out”. Field tests in magnesium deficiencies were due to excess phosphorus. *Magnesia phosphorica* in the potencies gave varied results depending on plant species treated.

APPEARANCE
Leaves yellow, bronze and redden and consequently are shredded. It is a fertile environment for mites, providing conditions in which they thrive.

All symptoms are worse in cold winds and draughts of cold air and rain. The plants thrive in heat, warm winds, and dry weather.

The roots may show bacterial canker with cracked epidermis. The cankers look red and raw. They do not readily take up water even though the plant is very thirsty. The capillaries may be paralysed; nutrients, sugars, starches and proteins are not transported to their correct places.

The leaves are yellow, bronze or red. They drop easily and the plant withers and dies. Photosynthesis is impaired due to lack of magnesium phosphate. All metabolic functions are impaired due to the inability to distribute phosphorus where it is needed.

The relationship between magnesium and phosphorus is a subject that has been overlooked by many soil and plant scientists. It is surmised that because magnesium is present in chlorophyll, there cannot be a problem. It forms the second most abundant element in animals, and is maybe the fifth major nutrient in plants. André Voisin and Dr. William Albrecht (quoted by Hylton, 1974,) have repeatedly warned that magnesium shortage would cause severe health problems for humans, animals, and plants. For more than 25 years, their warnings have been ignored. In the late 70s the USDA acknowledged the importance of magnesium in agriculture.

Without magnesium, phosphorus cannot be properly distributed in the cell nuclei, nor transported to other parts of the plant. A phosphorus deficiency cannot be rectified by any amount of phosphorus applied without magnesium. Thus, if the phosphorus content is to be increased, so must the magnesium. At the same time, excess phosphorus will render copper, potassium and zinc deficient.

RELATIONS

Compare: *Cuprum, Kali* preps, *Phosphorus*, *Zinc*.
Complementary: *Phosphorus Phosphoric acid Calcarea carbonica, Kali.*
Antidote to: *Phosphorus.*
Inimical: *Phosphorus, Cuprum, Kali, Zinc. Calcarea, Natrum.*
Antidoted by: *Manganum*.

Magnesia Sulphurica

Sulphate of magnesia. Epsom salts. $MgSO_4$. Trituration.

CLINICAL
Chlorosis of young leaves followed in later stages by total yellowing. Lodging, wilting, withering. Net blotch, blotches in general. Mildews. Damping off.

GENERAL
Magnesia sulphurica has more prostration than any other *Magnesia* preparation. Lodging of grains is commonly met by *Magnesia sulphurica*. Contrary to *Magnesia phosphorica,* the plant is excessively thirsty and the evaporation rate is very high. As described in the other *Magnesia* preparations, its relation to *Phosphorus* is very important. The sulphate content is responsible for the chlorosis and lodging, as lack of sulphate causes these symptoms. This does not mean that the sulphate component is the only reason. Magnesia has a relation to the content of phosphorus.

The roots are very dry with a rough epidermis. Contrary to *Magnesia phosphorica* conditions they readily take up water which evaporates almost immediately. It corresponds to diabetes in humans and the lack of sugars in the plant is a leading indication. Respiration and photosynthesis is impaired. Consequently all sugars stored in the roots will be used up causing weakness and lodging which shows in the yellowing of the young leaves. The plant is susceptible to net blotch and other blotches, and has a wilted appearance.

FLOWERS AND FRUITS
The flowers, which may come too early as the plant attempts to reproduce before it dies, are not productive; absence of pollen hinders fruit setting or prevents it altogether.

RELATIONS
Compare: *Phosphorus, Sulphur.*
Complementary: *Calcarea, Kali, Phosphorus, Phosphoricum acidum.*
Inimical: *Calcarea, Kali, Natrum Phosphoricum.*
Antidoted by: *Manganum.*

Manganum

Acetate of manganese. Manganum aceticum. $Mn(C_2H_3O_2)_2$. Solution. Carbonate of manganese. Manganum carbonicum. $MnCO_3$. Trituration.

CLINICAL
Chlorosis. Pale striping in barley, moulds, mildews, tan-spot, blotches and blights, wilting. Soil pH neutral or alkaline.

GENERAL
Manganese was isolated in the year Priestly discovered oxygen. Hahnemann introduced it into the materia medica and made provings with the acetate and carbonate. The symptoms of the two will be discussed together.

Manganese has a remarkable affinity for and in some respects resemblance to iron with which it is frequently found. The medicinal resemblance is very close. It has a similar capillary collapse to *Ferrum*, and *Calcarea fluoricum* with which it should be compared. Manganese is in plants an oxygen carrier. Plants cannot stand upright, wilting often and soon. The roots are congested and look pale. Many blotches and blights on the leaves as well as moulds and mildews. The plant requires little water. The flowers are affected in pollination with little or no pollen and incomplete fruit setting. Photosynthesis is impaired, capillary congestion and collapse, weak stems that break or bend too easily.

Manganese occurs in the *Alliums*, the *Cruciferae* and the *Cucurbitae*, as well as the *Solanacea*. *Natrum carbonicum*, although not the bicarbonate found in water, is worthy of comparison. Highly alkaline soils show more deficiency. Both *Natrum carbonicum*, and *Calcarea carbonica* must be studied in this connection. Because of a reduction in chlorophyll the photosynthetic capacity is impaired. The chlorosis begins pale green and can turn orange-red. Symptoms can appear both on the youngest and the oldest leaves dependent on the plant species.

Cabbage: general mottled yellow leaves. Beetroot: triangular leaves. This is known as 'speckled yellows'. (Hawson 1983) Onions and sweet corn have yellow stripes.

On acid soils liming can cause manganese deficiencies. The sulphate of lime is used in the crude form. ($MnSO_4$) Foliar spray can be used with much lower rates to be effective. Manganum is, therefore, best administered as a spray. It is best to spray the plants when still young, although equally good results can be obtained halfway through to maturity. Manganese is also used in a fungicide, eg Mancozeb. (Mason and Gartrell, undated.)

Manganese toxicity can be reduced by an application of *Silicea* The conclusion is that *Silicea* is the antidote to *Manganum.* It is also antidoted by *Kali*. If *Manganum* is deficient it increases susceptibility to take-all. Potassium excess can be inimical to *Manganum* thus increasing the susceptibility to take-all. (Brennan, 1991, 1992.)

External manifestations of Manganese deficiencies show as a gradual paling and faint yellowing between the veins. The yellowing is most prominent on older leaves. The interveinal areas finally become very yellow whilst the veins remain a dark green. (When younger leaves are affected, see *Zincum.*) The leaf shape remains normal. The colour is usually pale green (Zinc turns yellow). Shaded leaves more affected. Worse on loamy soils (Shorter and Cripps, 1985.) It occurs in all fruit growing districts. Manganese sulphate is usually used in a crude dose (500 g/100 l) to counteract this problem.

RELATIONS
Compare: *Kali permanganum.*
Complementary: *Ferrum.*
Inimical: *Calcarea carbonica, Kali, Phosphorus.*
Antidoted by: *Calcarea carbonica, Silicea, Kali.*
Antidote to: *Ferrum, Magnesia.*

Mentha Viridis/ Piperita/ Sativa spp.

Spearmint. Peppermint. NO *Labiatae*. Tincture of the whole plant.

CLINICAL
General pest control on the *Brassicae*. Fleas on livestock. Mice and rats. Ants, aphids, flea-beetles, mosquitoes, gnats, cabbage butterfly, caterpillar.

GENERAL
Grows on banks of river and damp watery places. *Mentha* is to respiratory problems what *Arnica* is to injuries and *Aconite* to inflammations. Singers will hold their voice when given *Mentha* shortly before their performance. As the bulk of the symptoms falls within the respiratory sphere it may prove to be of service in plants that suffer from acid rain (loss of leaves and needles gradual death of whole or forest). There are some concomitant spots, specks and blotches, while injuries cause rots.

The various species of mint have much in common and have been held in high medical esteem since ancient times. Cultivated mint is susceptible to disease itself. Grieve's herbal mentions that it is liable to attacks of rust which in her time was "incurable" (Grieve, 1931). From the homoeopathic viewpoint no disease is incurable provided the proper remedy is selected. *Aconite* or *Belladonna* can cure this disease. Although *Puccinia mentha*, the fungus responsible for rust in mint, is developed inside the plant, *Aconite* and *Belladonna* are taken up by the plant and can easily cure it. This is contrary to conventional agricultural chemicals which do not penetrate but are 'contact' sprays.

The various species of mint are effective in keeping pests off cabbage and other *Brassicae*. Another use for *Mentha* is the repelling of flies, mice and rats. In this capacity *Mentha* is to be used as a diluted essence.

The *Labiatae* all have healing properties for plants and as a family do much good in the garden. A more universal remedy combining the Labiatae into a single remedy is highly desirable for vegetables in general. Although mixtures of homoeopathic remedies are not used, it is only so with complexes as these are not made up of already potentised single substances. With new preparations mixing is done at the crude stage. Thus the whole plant of each species of Labiatae is mixed, out of which a mother-tincture is made. From this tincture potencies are prepared which deserve a separate proving. This is because many potentised substances antidote each other, especially so in the same natural order, especially in the complexes made up of already potentised substances. When mixed at tincture stage, before the potency is made, it should prove to be a remedy in its own right, much like *Hepar* (Hepar sulphuris calcareum), which is neither *Calcarea carbonica*, nor *Sulphur*, although providing symptoms pertaining to both.

Nasturtium

Tropeolum. NO *Crucifera*. Tincture of the seeds/whole plant.

CLINICAL
White aphids, squash bugs, white fly in tomatoes. Nematodes. Mealy bug.

GENERAL
Nasturtium is a companion plant that has the proven ability to protect other species against different species of aphids. Thus a homoeopathic dilution ought to be able to confer to plants a type of immunity to aphid infestation.

From experiments with plants it was noted that aphid infestation was only slightly influenced by Nasturtium in the 3x potency. More provings need to be conducted to establish with certainty the effects of the remedy. Experiments carried out on fennel infested with black aphid have been conducted. It deserves tests and provings on a larger variety of plants in different potencies.

Natrum Carbonicum

Sodium Carbonate. Common soda. Na_2CO_3. Trituration. Solution.

CLINICAL
Sterility. Chronic effects of sunstroke. Windburn. Blotch. Weak straggly plants. Eyespot. Black peach aphid. Bud worm. Citrus mite. Elephant weevil.

GENERAL
Natrum carbonica is the typical salt of the *Natrum* group. An excess of alkali burns off the superficial layers of the epidermis leaving the leaves dry and cracked. The roots are dry, sometimes mottled or ulcerated. The plant is excessively thirsty, whilst photosynthesis is impaired due to excess water stored in the plant. The flowers come too early resulting in sterility in cereals, and failure to form fruits in fruit producing plants. The plant is weak and cannot remain upright as in eyespot. The spots and blotches are blackish while the leaves dry out. Also tan-spot and halo-spot can be treated with this remedy. As these diseases have been described elsewhere, they have not been reproduced here.

FLOWERS AND FRUITS
Flowers appear prematurely. Sterility in cereals. Failure to form fruits.

WATER NEEDS
Excessive.

RELATIONS
Compare: *Kali* preparations.
Inimical: *Kali*.
Antidoted by: *Phosphorus.*

Natrum Muriaticum

Sodium chloride. Common salt. NaCl. Trituration. Solution.

CLINICAL
Scald, halo blight, stripe blight, salination, salt water bores, chlorosis.

GENERAL
If *Natrum carbonica* is the typical sodium salt, as *Kali carbonica* is of the potassium group, *Natrum muriaticum* is most important. "The problems of *Natrum muriaticum* may be regarded in a sense as the '*pons asinorum*' of homoeopathy. Those who can grasp, in a practical sense, the uses of this remedy will not meet with great difficulties elsewhere. Those who see nothing but common salt may conclude that they do not have the root of the matter in them." (Clarke.)

It may be inconceivable to some that the attenuations of *Natrum muriaticum* can act independently, whilst at the same time crude salt is applied in quantity, as is the case with many bores in the coastal regions. This problem is constantly confronting the homoeopath, and if he cannot master it he may not trouble his mind to try with other remedies.

As with all tissue salts, excess is antidoted or otherwise modified and negative effects are counteracted in an almost miraculous manner. A large number of plants in the coastal regions are steadily poisoned with quantities of salt water. Without restricting the quotient given, *Natrum muriaticum* 30x will antidote the effects of the crude. This has been repeatedly tested on turf in the coastal area of WA were salt-water bores are causing salination problems for bowling clubs. Good results have been obtained.

Schuessler adopted *Natrum muriaticum* from homoeopathy. Though arrived at by a different route, his indications are mostly identical to Hahnemann's.

"Water introduced to the plant through the roots, salty or not, enters through the epithelial cells by means of salt contained in these cells, for salt has the property of attracting water. Water is needed to moisten all tissues and cells. Every cell contains soda. The nascent chlorine which is split off the salt in the intracellular fluid combines with the soda. The sodium chloride arising from this combination attracts water. By this means the cell is enlarged and divides itself. Only in this way is growth through cell division possible. If there is no salt in the cells, then water remains in the intracellular fluid, and hydraemia results. The plant dries out, though it looks watery and bloated." (Schuessler, 1984.)

Common salt does not heal this problem since common cells can only receive salt in attenuated solutions. The salt is then redundant in the intracellular fluid and produces epidermical problems such as scald, halo blight and stripe blight where the tissue is waterlogged. Disturbances in the distribution of salt in cells produces residues that become transparent like water on the leaves.

"These are the theories of Schuessler, [altered by analogy in plants]. This theory is a useful means to string some characteristics of *Natrum muriaticum* together, but is by no means complete." (Clarke, 1990.)

Natrum muriaticum also corresponds to affections due to loss of fluids. *Natrum muriaticum* and *Kali muriaticum* are related and correspond in plant nutrition. *Kali muriaticum* can greatly reduce the effects of salt-water bores. These two remedies should be carefully compared. The nutrient functions in plants can be adversely affected when an imbalance between the two occurs in a plant. Either can have an excess or a deficiency.

The type of irrigation and its frequency as well as the water quality have great influence on plant nutrient levels. (Ojala et al. 1983, Stark et al. 1983, Feigin 1985, Cerda and Martinez 1988)

The capillary system is disturbed resulting in chlorosis, which in turn affects photosynthesis and protein levels. Capillaries are congested and constricted. No matter how much NPK is given the plants emaciate and become weak. Plants are very thirsty, especially after salt water from bores. Also it increases cadmium uptake.

FLOWERS AND FRUITS

The flowers produce no pollen and fruit setting is impaired. Pollen may also be too abundant too early. Waterlogged areas on stems and leaves. Imperfect assimilation of nutrients.

APPEARANCE

Thin emaciated plants, despite repeated fertilisation. Flowers produce no pollen, or too early production of pollen. Salt damage due to salt water bores. Salination problems. Black peach aphid.

RELATIONS

Compare: *Kali.*

Complementary: *Kali muriaticum.*

Antidoted by: *Kali muriaticum, Phosphorus.*

Antidote to: *Natrum muriaticum*, most nutrients.

Inimical: *Kali.*

Natrum Phosphoricum

Phosphate of soda. Na_2HPO_4.

CLINICAL
Stripe rust, leaf rust, photosynthesis problems, banana rust thrips.

GENERAL
Natrum phosphoricum is found in the sap, the cells of the cambium, and the intercellular fluids. Through the action of *Natrum phosphoricum*, carbonic acid is formed. *Natrum phosphoricum* is able to bind itself to carbonic acid, receiving two parts of carbonic acid for each part of phosphoric acid. When it has thus bound the carbonic acid it conveys it to the leaves. The oxygen taken up in photosynthesis liberated the carbonic acid which is only loosely bound to the phosphoric acid. The carbonic acid is then exhaled and exchanged for oxygen which is absorbed by iron and manganese in the sap. During the day this process is reversed. It is obvious that *Natrum phosphoricum* is the remedy par excellence for problems with photosynthesis. It can be used for rusts, and indeed in all cases where the leaves develop a golden yellow scab. It must be compared with *Aconite*.

The normal relation of antidote is here totally suspended. *Phosphorus* has here the action of a complement. In this way certain features of a remedy may be totally altered. What normally is a particular feature of a remedy can completely disappear. Although partaking of features of *Natrum* and *Phosphorus*, this is a very different remedy with its own particulars.

RELATIONS
Compare: *Aconite, Carbolic acid, Ferrum, Manganum, Phosphorus.*
Complementary: *Carbolicum acidum, Phosphoric acidum.*
Inimical: *Kali.*

Natrum Salicylicum

Salicylate of sodium. $NaC_7H_5O_3$. Trituration, solution.

CLINICAL
Tobacco mosaic virus, blue mould, anthracnose, downy mildew, angular leaf spot, potato virus, alfalfa virus, barley yellow dwarf virus, aphid.

GENERAL
Salicylic acid is found in nature in the leaves and bark of willows, in oil of wintergreen, and is synthetically obtained from carbolic acid. Recent research has shown that aspirin greatly speeds recovery when given to sick plants. It has also been shown to be effective as a food preservative. Prolonged use in humans causes Ménières disease (auditory nerve vertigo), gastric disturbances, delirium, septicaemia and necrosis of the tibia. These symptoms in humans can point us to some indications for its use in plants. Roots may be covered with white or red patches. Many pustules, pale or brown on the leaves. Septoria blotch, tan spot, ring spot, eye spot, scald and all other blotches and mosaic viruses may improve under *Salicylic acid* regardless of plant species.

Plants defective in lime salts which often wilt easily and do not hold upright well. The sap is not of normal consistency, it looks and feels as though it is decaying. There is capillary congestion and imbalance in nutrient uptake. Plants become infected and die.

Hydroponic testing has been under way since 1992 by Malany, Klessig, Pierpoint and Vernooy et. al. Their results show only crop resistance through "inoculation". They do not signify cures. From these results inference may be drawn as to possible cures. The *Salicylic acid* remedy, being homoeopathic, is different from the crude form used during the tests, and will prove to be less aggressive and thus may take longer to produce results in provings. Plants have their own immune system. *Salicylic acid* affects other plant processes also. Foliar application has shown to speed up and increase flowering, adventitious root initiation, and fruit yield. It increases absorption of *Kali* and reduces germination of lettuce seed.

RELATIONS
Compare: *Silicea, Ferrum phosphoricum, Phosphorus, Calcarea fluorica, Salicylic acid.*
Inimical: *Kali.*
Antidoted by: *Phosphorus.*

Natrum Sulphuricum

Sodium Sulphate. Na_2SO_4. Trituration, solution.

CLINICAL
Waterlogging, photosynthesis impaired. Destruction of leaf tissue, leaves turn yellow, stunted plants, chlorosis, ergot, rusts, aphids, banana rust thrips.

GENERAL
Sodium sulphate was discovered by Glauber in 1658 and is still known as Glauber's salt. Grauvogl describes the character of those needing the homoeopathic equivalent as a state in which there is extreme sensitiveness to damp, rain and waterlogging, or growth near bodies of standing water, such as dams or lakes.

The action of *Natrum sulphuricum* is contrary to that of the chloride. Both attract water but for different reasons; *Natrum muriaticum* takes up water destined to split up cells necessary for growth. *Natrum sulphuricum* attracts the water formed during the retrogressive metamorphosis of cells and eliminates it from the system. It draws water from the superannuated serum cells causing their destruction. *Natrum sulphuricum* stimulates the epithelial cells in the capillaries thus eliminating superfluous water from the system. If the activities of sodium sulphate are disturbed, the elimination of superfluous water is disturbed and hydraemia is the result. *Natrum sulphuricum* is indicated in plants that are too rich in water, are always worse in damp conditions, and get better when the weather is dry and warm.

The roots are dry whilst the plant is thirsty. They have a dirty green/grey or green/brown appearance from moulds. Through the yellowing of the leaves there is impaired photosynthesis, with the resulting low protein content.

Drying out with waterlogging is a typical *Natrum sulphuricum* feature. Many rusts are favoured by this condition (see *Aconite, Belladonna*). Some blotches require wet conditions for their development.

FLOWERS AND FRUITS
Flowers are affected, but no reports of crop loss or failure to fruit have been recorded. In general it can be said that any disease that is caused by drying out of plants in moist conditions, particularly when the water is excessive, can greatly benefit from *Natrum sulphuricum.*

As with all tissue salts, these remedies require very careful monitoring, absolute minimum dose, and caution in prescription.

RELATIONS
Compare; *Aconite, Belladonna.*
Inimical: *Kali.*
Antidoted by: *Phosphorus.*

Nitricum Acidum

Nitric acid. Aqua fortis. Strong water. HNO_3 solution.

CLINICAL
Nitrogenous rich soils and plants. Phosphorus excess. Blotch, black point, mildew, eyespot, purpling of stem and leaves.

GENERAL
When strong Nitric acid comes in contact with the epidermis, it destroys the upper layers and turns them yellow, but as the protein coagulates it forms a barrier against its own action. It regulates the excess uptake of phosphorus as well as nitrogen. It is one of the chief antidotes to mercury. In soils where mercury poisoning is detected plants can be safely grown provided a dose of *Nitric acidum* is administered soon after planting to prevent the uptake of mercury in the plant. *Nitric acidum* follows *Kali carbonicum* in photosynthesis problems, such as deficient chlorophyll.

Nitric acidum acts on the roots, the flowers, especially the stamen, the bark, which fissures and cracks, the leaves, creating problems in photosynthesis.

At the 2-4 leaf stage chlorosis may appear. The midriffs turn pink, as well as the petioles. Later the stems turn purple or red. The older leaves turn yellow to orange-red, with red veins. The leaves die and gradually the whole plant becomes affected. As a consequence there is a reduction in branching. (Mason and Gartrell undated)

The roots have dark blotches or green (except legumes). They usually have an offensive smell. They are swollen and have an ulcerated appearance. The plant craves lime or alkaline substances.

The stem is either too rigid or too weak, and both are indications of excess nitrogen and phosphorus. The latter affects the flowers and stamen which either pollinate too early or not at all. Fruiting is thus affected and crop loss may result. (See *Kali Nitricum*)

APPEARANCE
Purpling of underside of leaves, pink/red. Yellowing of leaves (also in nitrogen deficiency). Bark cracks, (except on eucalypts, for example, where bark is shed as a normal feature). Bark fissures.

RELATIONS
Nitrogen fixation in beans and peas may be affected by a lack of molybdenum.
Complementary: *Molybdenum, Nitricum acidum.*
Follows *Kali carbonicum*.
Antidote to: *Molybdenum*.

Ocymum Minimum / Basilicum

Basil. NO *Labiatae*. Tincture of the whole plant.

CLINICAL
All pests and diseases of tomatoes. Anthracnose, bacterial cancer, bud worm, fusarium wilt, russet mite, spotted wilt, tobacco mosaic virus, blossom end rot. Flies. Mosquitoes. Tomato mite. Red-legged earth mite. Two-spotted mite.

GENERAL
Basil, as a companion plant, protects tomatoes from both pests and diseases "almost as if giving them a wrap-around shield" (Hylton 1974). For those who grow tomatoes as a commercial crop, and who have little space in which companion planting is impractical, homoeopathic remedies can solve the problem.

Thus, bacterial canker, fusarium wilt, spotted wilt, mosaic virus and blossom end rot, can all be treated with *Ocymum*. It may not be suited to treat other plants because it is a companion plant to tomatoes.

Ocymum is a constitutional remedy for tomatoes because of its special affinity. In companion plants this phenomenon is frequently met with, and can provide new insights in the relationships between the different remedies in the context of human treatment. From further study much can be learned about the internal relations between many different remedies that to date have not enjoyed such extensive scrutiny.

Other varieties of *Ocymum*, like *Ocymum* canum, and *Ocymum* gratissimum are equally efficacious and may be substituted for *Ocymum minimum* in their native countries, such as India, Japan, Indonesia, Malaysia, Persia and Africa, or South America. It will also improve the taste of the tomato crop.

Oxalic Acid

Hydrogen oxalate, $C_2H_2O_4$. Trituration or tincture.

CLINICAL
Respiratory insufficiency.

GENERAL
Respiration in plants is designated as the Krebs cycle. *Oxalic acid* plays an important role in this cycle which involves a series of chemical changes in which *Citricum acid, Acetic acid,* and *Oxalic acid* all play an approximately equal role.

The importance of *Oxalic acid* in respiratory problems, such as cell collapse and symptoms such as chlorosis, cannot be underestimated. *Oxalic acid* will act in cases where the acids are imperfectly functioning (only discernible when laboratory tests are conducted). These tests must focus on the levels of CO_2 production and the uptake of oxygen. A deficient uptake of oxygen indicates and defines this issue.

Oxalic acid is seen as an organ remedy of the first order. Together with *Acetic acid* and *Citric acid* it can be seen in a similar vein as the trio of Kent or Hahnemann's three miasmatic remedies. This comparison is somewhat poor, but it conveys the general idea.

RELATIONS
Antidoted by: *Calcarea carbonica, Magnesia.*
Compare: *Acetic acid, Citric acid, Kali oxalicum, Phosphoric acidum, Sulphur.*

Phosphorus

The element phosphorus - P. Phosphorus-saturated solution in absolute alcohol. Trituration of red amorphous phosphorus.

CLINICAL
Fruit-spotting bug, fruit piercing moth. Halo-stripe, stripe blight, scald, impaired photosynthesis, necrosis, engorgement of the leaves, chlorosis with smaller leaves than usual in either excess or lack of phosphorus. Droopy appearance, weak plants, rusts, blotches, dry leaf problems, dry rots, soft rots, aphids, banana rust thrips, dried fruit beetle, fruit fly.

GENERAL
Phosphorus, (light bearer, morning star) was discovered in 1673 by Brandt, an alchemist of Hamburg, and shortly afterwards by Kunkil in Saxony. Teste informs us that immediately afterwards attempts were made to use it in medicine. Kunkil made it into his "Luminous Pills".

Phosphorus has been called the 'master key to agriculture', because low crop production is more often due to a deficiency of this element than of any other nutrient. Deficiencies show up differently in different plants; in cereals the leaves turn purplish, legumes become bluish green and stunted. Most plants, however, turn dark green with red or purple tints.

Waterlogging increases phosphorus availability in the soil. Also, plant life affects the pH and the availability of nutrients. Plants can change the soil environment and its level of alkalinity or acidity. The occurrence of barley grass is correlated to the concentrations of organic calcium, transfer of nutrients and the presence of NH_4, available phosphorus, exchangeable cations and soluble salts. (Metson et al. 1971.)

High soil concentrations of phosphorus are also connected with perennial ryegrass causing ryegrass toxicity in sheep. When potassium was increased the ryegrass responded with an equal increase, while a low level of potassium reduced the occurrence of ryegrass in the paddock, while Paspalum and brown top bent increased.

Sheep sorrel, which is supposed to grow on acid soils, actually makes the soil more alkaline. It is an acid soil pioneer plant, which prepares the soil for plants which require a more alkaline soil.

Both too much and too little phosphorus can cause changes in pest behaviour. An imbalance encourages egg production in spider mites, as mentioned by the USDA. Deficiency can lead to problems with whitefly in the field and in potting mixes. In field tests mixed results were obtained, depending on the plant species and the potting mix used.

Phosphorus and iron interaction must always be considered when dealing with phosphorus imbalances. Phosphorus is an important element for enzyme binding in the Krebs Cycle. A deficiency shows in discolouration of the leaves and stems to dark blue-green. Stunted growth, reduced quantity and quality of the seeds and fruits are the most observable symptoms. Increased senescence and abscission are marked. (Bolland, 1978.)

Phosphorus sources in agriculture consist of mono-calcium phosphate, calcium phosphate and sodium phosphate.

Phosphorus is also found in organo-phosphates which are used as pesticides. It has been evident that the re-emergence of pests can be triggered by the use of pesticides, particularly aphids as they like high phosphorus environments. Similarly, herbicides like 2,4D can make plants susceptible to pest and blight attack. This is because herbicides have a damaging effect on any plant. (Ingratta and Brown, 1981). Thus the whole edifice of chemical farming stands or falls on the premise that chemical fertilisers, pesticides, and herbicides do not negatively affect the crop. Yet residues of poisonous substances will be found on almost any type of food crop. The "allowable amount of residue" is stipulated by the "Clean Foods Act". Most chemical agricultural agents have a withholding period to allow most of the poisons to run off before it is allowed on the market. Organo-phosphates have a particular feature; they have a short half life which means that they break down rather fast.

Oedematous spots in leaves as in halo blight and stripe blight. Photosynthesis is impaired. Generally all diseases where the plants show watery cells and their concomitant problems.

Phosphorus is an excellent remedy for the effects of lead poisoning, seen so often on road verges both in the city and in the country.

Plants appear sallow and bloated. Flowers appear premature with excess phosphorus. *Phosphorus* given shortly before flowering causes increased flowering and thus leads to greater yields.

Phosphorus profoundly affects the nutrition and function of every tissue, notably the hardest (cambium and bark) and the softest (flowers and fruits). It causes an increase in growth whilst continuous use later causes degeneration.

The plant is very thirsty and wilts easily in dry spells. As can be seen from *Natrum phosphoricum*, it has a great affinity for photosynthesis and respiration. The leaves can be totally congested and capillary action paralysed, resulting in the collapse of the entire plant. When phosphorus is in excess, the process as depicted under *Natrum phosphoricum* becomes untenable, because the carbonic acid cannot keep up with the phosphoric acid which is bound to oxygen to form the acid. As oxygen is attracted to hydrogen, water is the result and waterlogging takes place in the leaves. This restricts photosynthesis and ultimately leads to total capillary system collapse.

The roots have shrivelled skins which feel as though they are loose around the core of the root. Very dry; yellow with a brown core. The plant is very thirsty, yet no nutrient is taken up as the plant already has an excess nutrient and suffers from ill health as a consequence.

FLOWERS AND FRUITS

The flowers are abundant and fruits are big with tough skins, but they have a watery interior and little taste. When there is excess phosphorus, flowers come too early and fail to fully develop the stamen. Sterility is the result. The reproduction is sublime if *Phosphorus* is given at the right time.

APPEARANCE

The diseases connected with *Phosphorus* are similar to *Natrum phosphoricum* and *Kali phosphoricum* but more pronounced. Dry rots are similar to *Calcarea, Silicea, Calcarea fluorica* or *Lapis albus*. Soft rots, Armillaria root rots, collar rot citrus, bacterial soft rot, to name but a few examples.

Armillaria root rot. (*Armillaria* spp). Leaves may turn brown around edges, or they may yellow and fall. Wilting and dieback are common. Citrus may set a very healthy fruit crop in spring but collapses in the dry, hot summer.

The roots have a white sheath of fungal hyphae in or under the epidermis, which smells strongly of mushrooms. The woody part is either dry and powdery, or wet and jelly like. Long shoelace like structures are typical and help spread from root to root and tree to tree.

The fungus is a weak parasite on native trees. It grows on old roots and stumps, spreading from there. In fall when weather is humid and soil is moist, yellowish brown toadstools grow up from the rotted roots and appear on the soil surface. Plants affected: woody ornamentals and smaller plants like strawberries, and many fruit trees.

Bacterial soft rot. (*Erwina carotovora*). The bacteria that cause this affliction are very common in soil, or on plants. They prefer succulent plants. In damp weather they cause the most trouble. Also plants recovering from pest attack or other disease are prone to soft rot. The rot is always soft and foetid-smelling with a slimy appearance.

On potatoes, the first symptoms are soft depressed areas around lenticels. It is easy to distinguish from gangrene by the peculiar softness. On calla lilies, the disease starts below the ground. Water-soaked areas appear at the bottom of flower and leaf stalks which rot and fall over.

Sweet corn has a similar picture; the stem just above the soil becomes water-soaked, dark brown and slimy; it collapses. Carrots and potatoes are contaminated at harvest time and rot in storage.

Plants affected:
Fleshy parts of succulent plants, roots, tubers, fleshy leaf bases, fruit buds, and stem, crucifers, potatoes, celery, lettuce, ornamentals, irises, dahlias and calla lilies.

Collar rot - citrus (*Phytophthora citropthora*). This disease is caused by a fungus which inhabits the soil and is only active in certain conditions. When the leaves go yellow and the tree looks unhealthy it might have collar rot.

The first sign is gum oozing out of the bark near ground level. After some time, the bark may look wet. Still later, it becomes dry, brittle and split. If not treated the rot will ring bark the tree. It grows only in damp conditions when waterlogged or when vegetables or weeds have been allowed too close to the trunk.

Plants affected:
This list begins with the most susceptible and ends with the most resistant. Eureka and Lisbon lemons, Washington navel grapefruit, Valencia rootstock and mandarins. Trifoliata, Citrauge, Troyer and Carrizo are completely resistant.

RELATIONS
Compare: *Ferrum.*
Antidote to: *Lead poisoning. Natrums.*
Inimical: *Alum., Calcarea, Ferrum, Magnesia, Manganum, Zinc.*

Porcellio

Common slater. *Porcellio scaber*. NO *Isopoda*. Trituration of the live insect.

CLINICAL
Slaters, pillbugs, sowbugs, cellar worms.

GENERAL
Clarke has a remedy called *Oniscus* which, from the description, appears to be the same as *Porcellio*.

Adult slaters are between 9-15 mm long, oval in shape and fairly flat. There are grey, brown, and pink varieties, depending on age. They feed on organic matter, chewing the stems and cotyledons of seedlings. They can be serious pests.

Excellent control was achieved for up to three months from a single dose of the freshly prepared 6x potency.

RELATIONS
Compare: *Cantharis*.

Ricinus Communis

Castor oil plant. Palma christi. NO *Euphorbiaceae*. Tincture or trituration of fresh seeds or fresh plant.

CLINICAL
Pests in viticulture: vine mite, rust mite, grapevine moth, hawk moth, scale. Pests in *Cucurbitae*. Worms.

GENERAL
This plant is a native of India. From Clarke's Materia Medica we can learn that the leaves of this plant have an especially powerful effect on the breast and the generative sphere. From this fact one can deduce the action on the flowers and fruits on plants. As it is a good companion to grapevines its action on grape flowers and fruits is borne out by the provings. As with all plant pest and disease remedies, analogy is the most often used means of determining its effects on plants. Subsequent provings usually - but by no means always - confirm the analogy. Sometimes, however, it proves to have additional features not arrived at through analogy, but either through clinical experience or provings.

From the Materia Medica it has become clear that it acts as a vermifuge. However, it needs to be used with caution, as too high a dose can severely purge the animal and debilitate it to a great extent. Analogous is its action on nematodes.

Ruta

Rue. NO *Rutaceae*. Ruta graveolens. Tincture of the whole plant.

CLINICAL
Pip or croup in fowls, flies and other pests. Rabies. Excessive pollination and diminished fruit setting.

GENERAL
Grows at the border of moist meadows and in ditches. Rue is such a powerful irritant that the species *Ruta montana* is even dangerous to handle with gloves. Since ancient times it has been used as a remedy against rabies, as well as pip and croup in fowl. It was the favourite of the Prophet Mohammed, because it cured him of a disease which no other herb could cure.

Because of its action in the crude, causing pollination and fruit setting problems, it will cure these in the potencies. Thus its action is similar to *Silicea*, but presents its own set of symptoms.

Besides the obvious insect repelling qualities of *Ruta*, it affects the flowers in a most peculiar way - it causes excessive pollination while at the same time it diminishes fruit setting to almost nil. This may account for the fact other plants do not thrive in the vicinity of rue.

This remedy was not yet used on plants but good results were obtained from its use on dogs suffering from flies!

Salicylic Acid

$C_6H_4(OH)COOH$. Artificially prepared from phenol.

CLINICAL
Potato virus. Tobacco mosaic virus, blue mould anthracnose, downy mildew, angular leaf spot, Pseudomonas infections.

GENERAL
Salicylic acid forms an important part in the immune system of plants. Without it the plant can do little to fight off diseases or pests. When plants are invaded by a pathogen a number of responses may be induced in the area surrounding the infection. These responses include rapid cell death to prevent the spread of the disease, while healthy cell walls are strengthened and antimicrobial agents are released. The unaffected parts develop more resistance to further infections by either viral, bacterial, or fungal pathogens.

This mode of resistance is termed 'systemic acquired resistance'. These mechanisms have been recognised since the early part of this century, but little is known about the 'how' of this response. Evidently there must be some messenger substance that provokes the healthy cells to action. Salicylic acid has been implicated as a component (Vernooy et al. 1994. "The Plant Cell".)

Salicylic acid is not the translocated signal, but is required in signal transduction. In a similar manner as a vaccination works in humans, there are now voices that demand "plant vaccination". However if it is not broken don't fix it, as the saying goes. In an infected leaf, salicylic acid accumulates at the site of infection. When salicylic acid is not available to plants the systemic acquired resistance does not work. In addition, when *Salicylic acid* has been given, it shows increased resistance buildup. Most research has concentrated on tobacco mosaic virus. Only a small number of diseases and crops have been studied. Further testing is certainly warranted but, in this case, with potencies of *Natrum salicylicum* and *Salicylic acid* which is considered under a separate heading in this book.

APPEARANCE
Several different viruses cause mosaic symptoms on potatoes and other related plants. These are referred to as potato virus X, A and Y. Symptoms vary from a light mottling of yellow and green on the leaves, to yellow spots or crinkling of leaf tissue. Sometimes veins may blacken and plants die early.

Mosaic virus attacks many plants. On cabbage, cauliflower, and broccoli, the first symptoms are yellow rings on the youngest leaves later turning mottled, with rings and blotches of different shades of green. In warm weather this is the case. In cold weather, black rings appear on the older leaves.

(Continued on page 140)

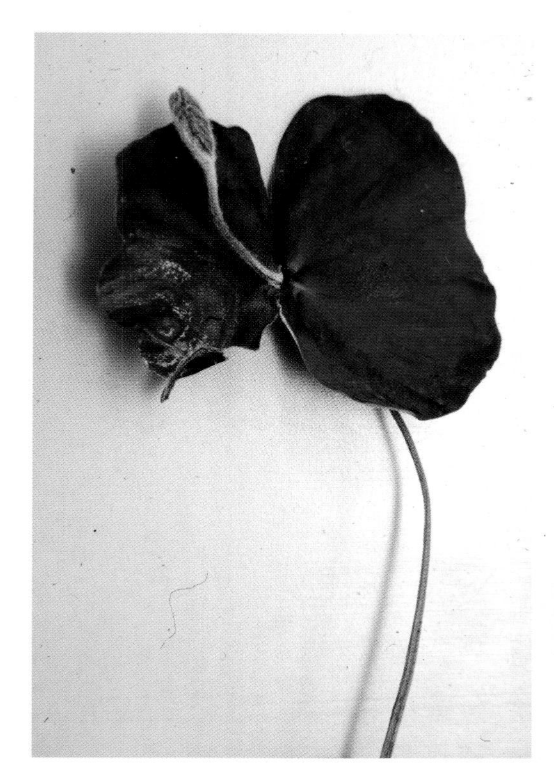

The challenge of finding the best remedy is balanced by the reward. A single application can protect a plant throughout a season, sometimes beyond. Therefore, one would like to spot signs of stress early in a plant's life. A particularly attractive prospect would be to treat seeds - see *Silicea* on page 146. The biodynamic preparations have been used as seed baths for many years, and Dr Murthy in India has achieved success in forestalling disease at this first stage.

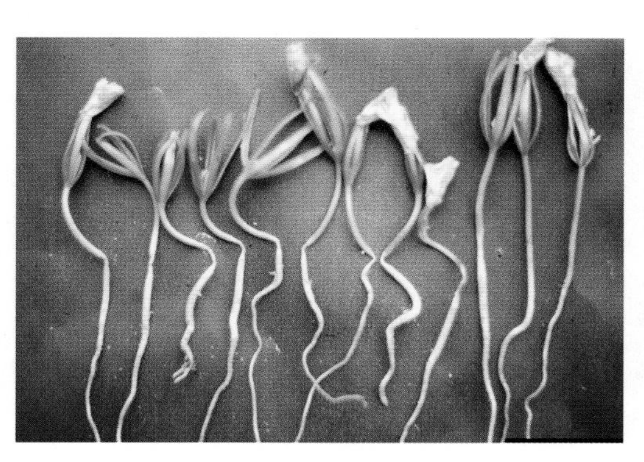

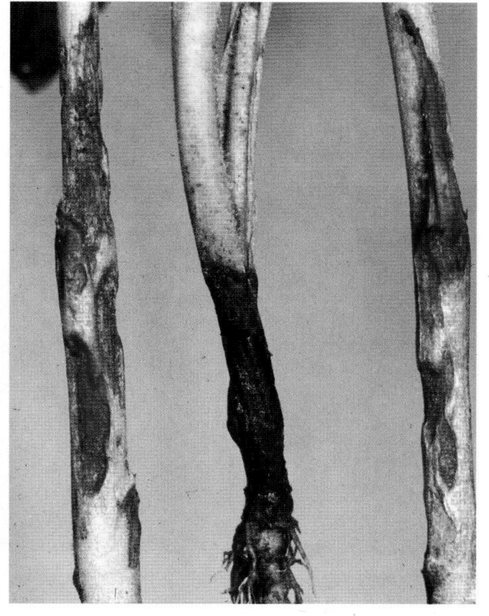

For seedlings and younger plants, 'damping off' has been successfully negotiated using *Calc., Carbo v., Cham., Mag.c., Mag.s.* Puny young plants have been strengthened by *Silicea*, and plants have been brought back from the brink with *Carbo veg.*

However, many signs of stress manifest at the later leaf stages and observing, differentiating, and diagnosing is crucial for selecting the right remedy. The following pages show a small variety of visual symptoms on leaves which have been addressed by homoeopathic remedies.

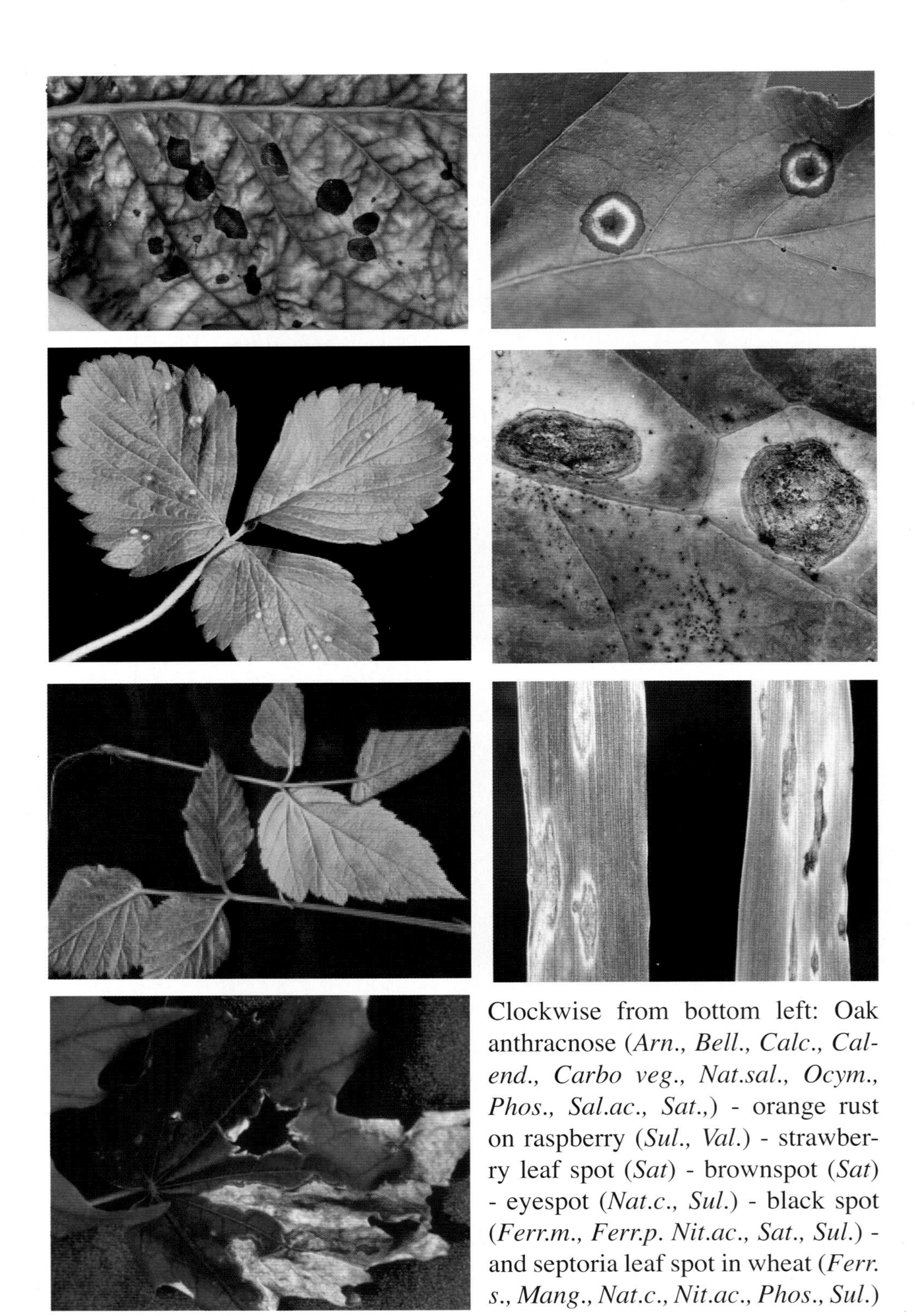

Clockwise from bottom left: Oak anthracnose (*Arn., Bell., Calc., Calend., Carbo veg., Nat.sal., Ocym., Phos., Sal.ac., Sat.,*) - orange rust on raspberry (*Sul., Val.*) - strawberry leaf spot (*Sat*) - brownspot (*Sat*) - eyespot (*Nat.c., Sul.*) - black spot (*Ferr.m., Ferr.p. Nit.ac., Sat., Sul.*) - and septoria leaf spot in wheat (*Ferr. s., Mang., Nat.c., Nit.ac., Phos., Sul.*)

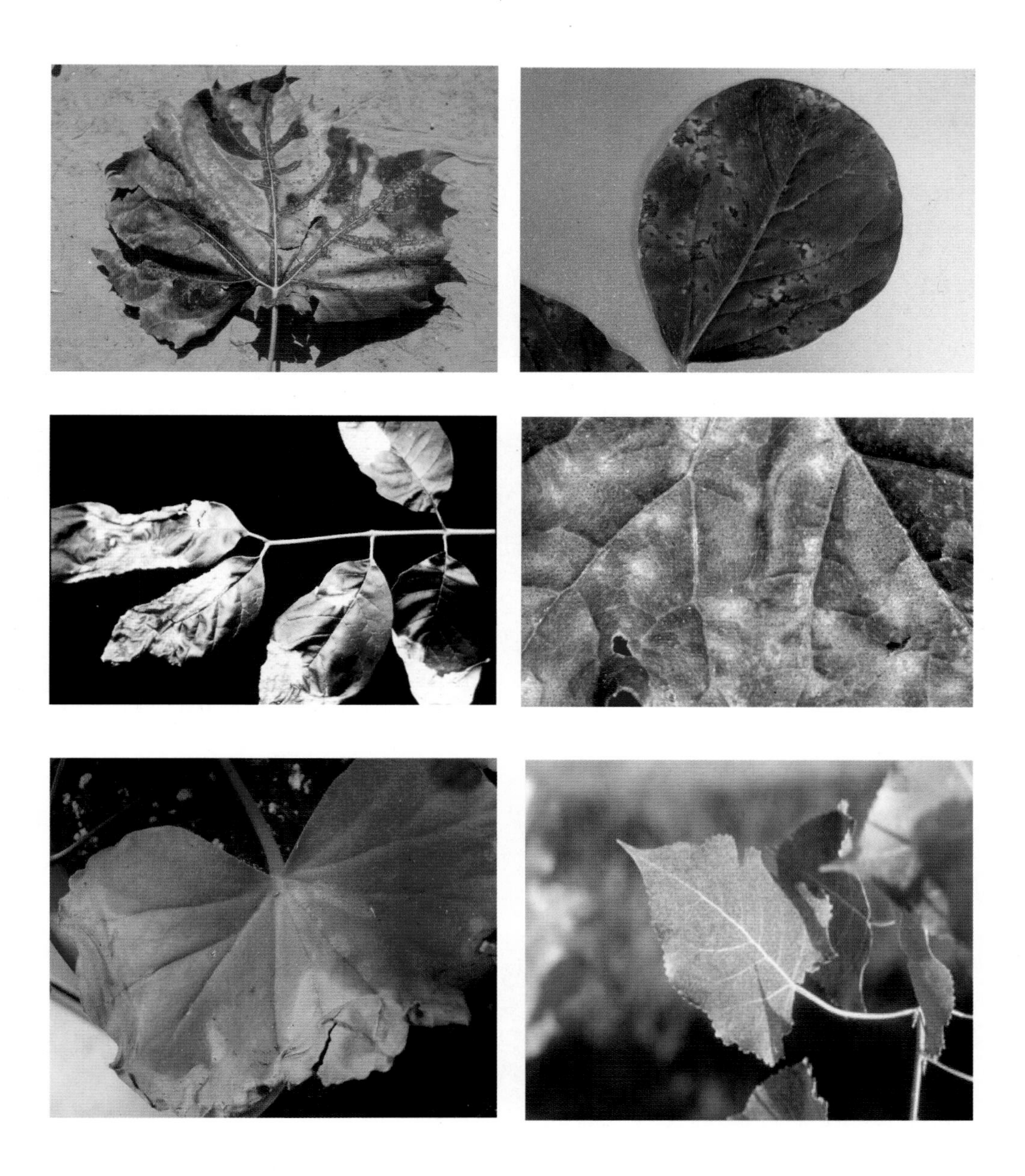

Clockwise from above left: Bacterial wilt (*Ocym., Sat.*) - Anthracnose in ash (*Arn., Bell., Calc., Calend., Carbo v., Nat.sal., Ocym., Phos., Sal.ac., Sat.*) - Bacterial leaf scorch in sycamore *(Mag. carb*) - bacterial blight (*Ferr.m., Ferr.p., Hyssop., Lact.ac., Nat.sal., Ocym., Phos., Sal.ac., Sat., Sul.*) - downy mildew on melon (*All.c., Calc.p. Ferr.s., Kali m., Kali perm., Lact.ac., Mag. s. Nit.ac., Sul.*) - rust on poplar (*Acon., Bell.*)

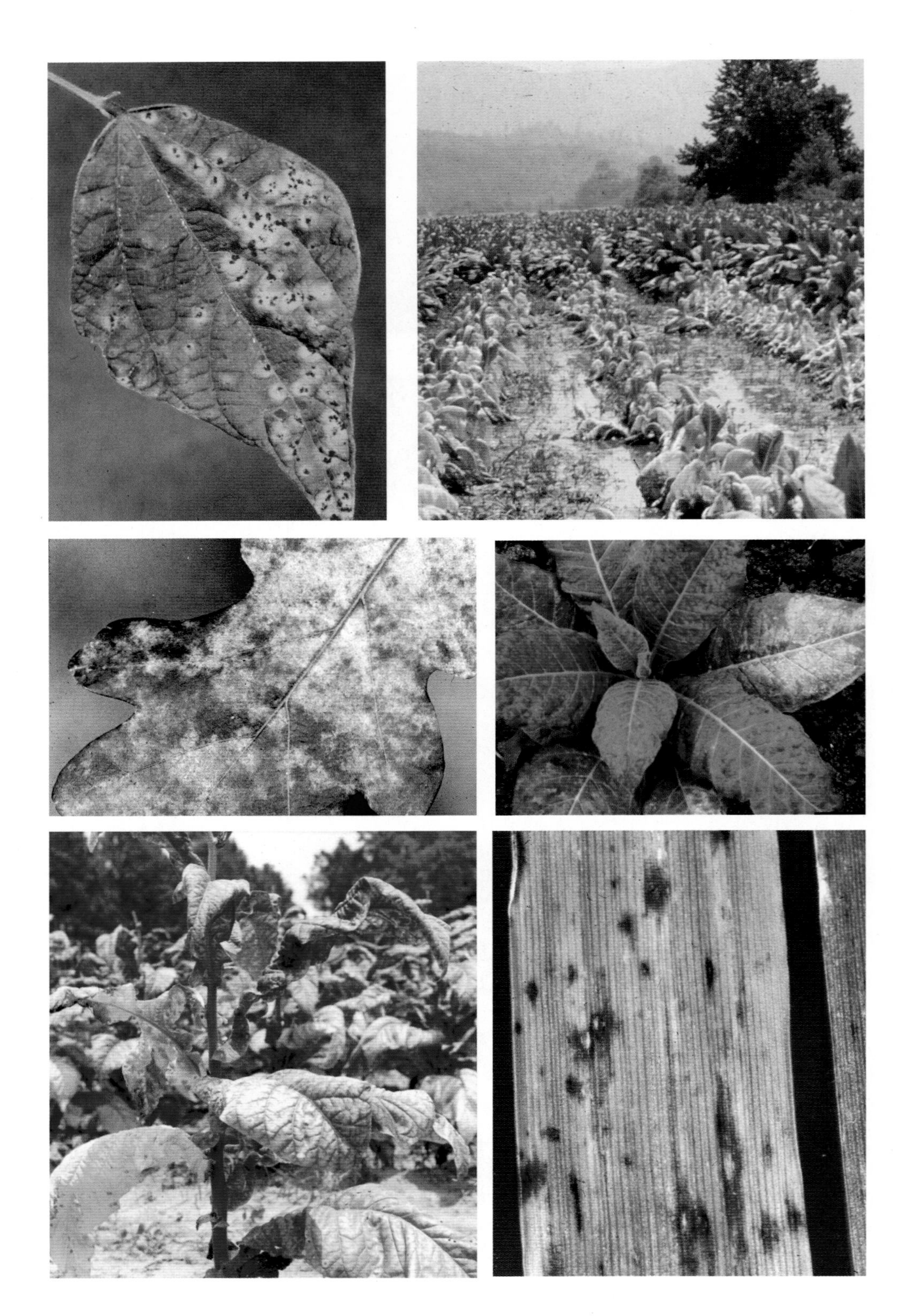

Opposite page - clockwise from bottom left: Fusarium on tobacco (*Ocym., Sat.*) - powdery mildew on oak (*All.c., Equis., Ferr.s., Kali m., Kali perm., Lact.ac., Mag.s., Nit.ac., Sil., Sul.*) - bean rust (*Acon., Amm.carb., Bell., Berb., Canth., Ferr.m., Ferr.p. Nat.sul., Phos., Sat., Sul.*) - the effects of waterlogging on tobacco (*Mag.p., Mag.s., Nat.c., Nat.m., Nat.sul., Val.*) - tobacco mosaic virus (*Lact.ac., Lapis, Nat.sal. Ocym., Sal.ac.*) - and leaf blotch on oat (*Calc.fl.. Calc.p., Mag.s., Mang., Nat.c., Nit.ac., Phos., Sul.*)

If the stress is not sufficiently manifest until the plant sets fruit, a reliable diagnosis can only be made later. Below, clockwise from bottom left, we see the effects of loose smut on barley (*Ustil.*), botrytis or grey mould on strawberries (*Ferr.s., Kali m., Sul.*), nematode on wheat (*Calend., Calc.fl., Calc.p., Carbo v., Nast., Sul., Tanac., Teuc. Val. Zinc m*) and corn smut (*Ustil.*).

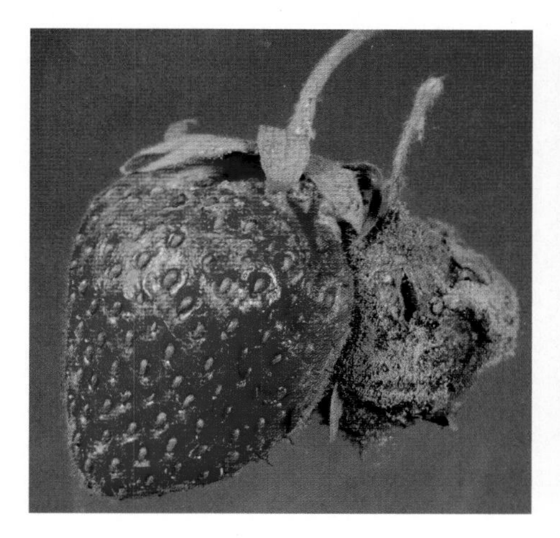

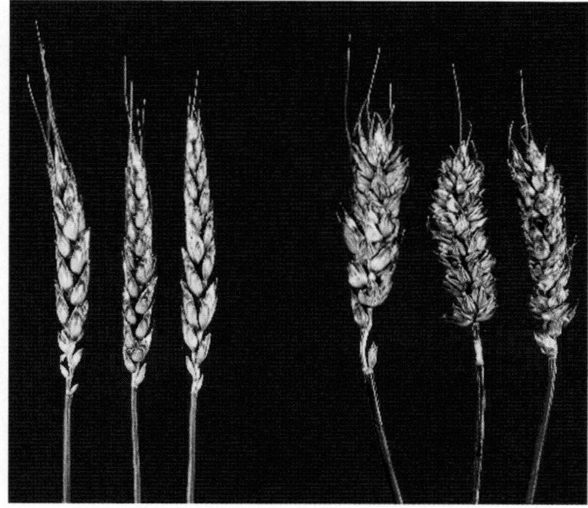

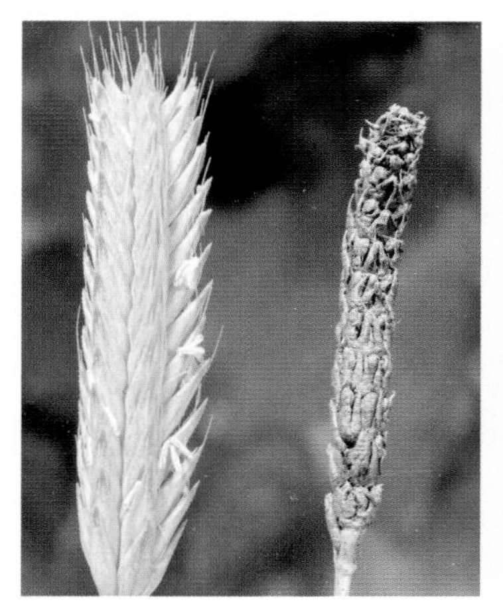

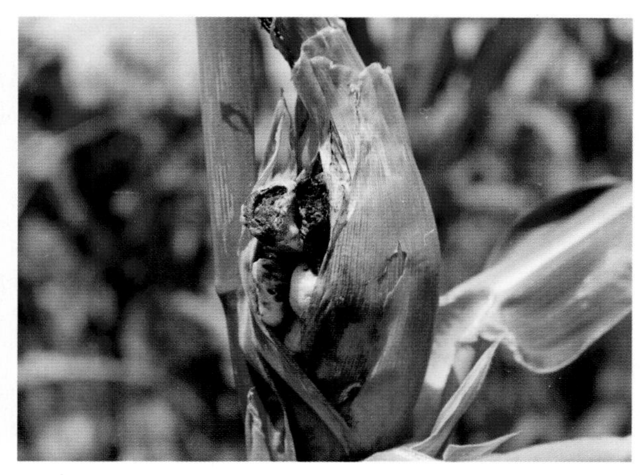

When pests get out of balance, homoeopathy has been found to help. Clockwise from right: Tobacco bud worm (*All.c., Bombyx., Car., Samb., Sil., Staphyl., Syrph., Tanac.*) - two spot spider mite (*Coccin., Ocym., Sul.*) - the pupae of the diamondback moth (*Aran., Bombyx., Caribida., Coccin. Samb., Staphyl., Syrph., Tanac.*) - the asparagus beetle (*Calend.*) - and the squash bug (*Nast., Staphylinida, Syrphidia.*) Note: I have created the last two remedies from predators that are used in IPM.

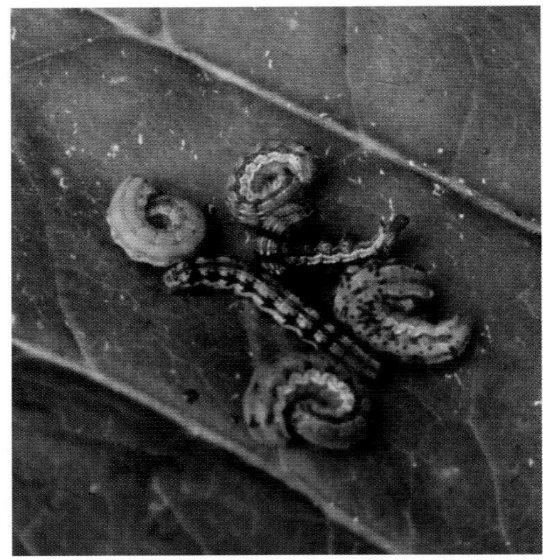

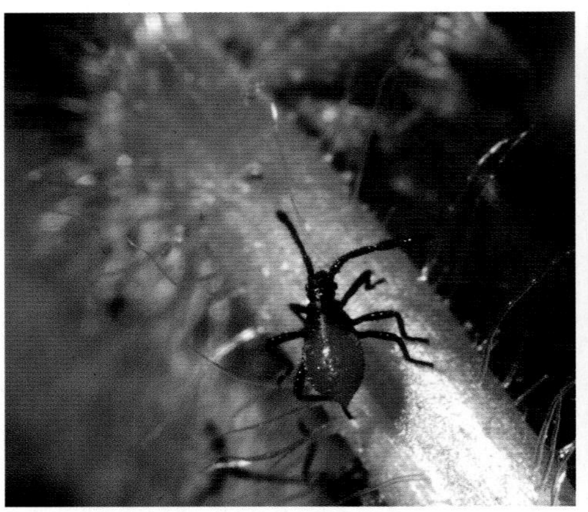

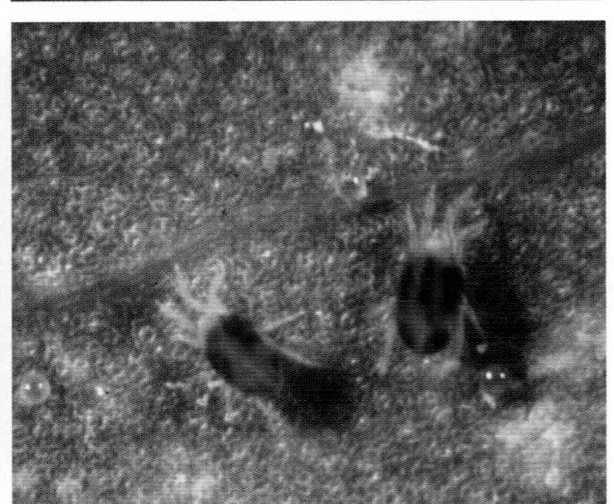

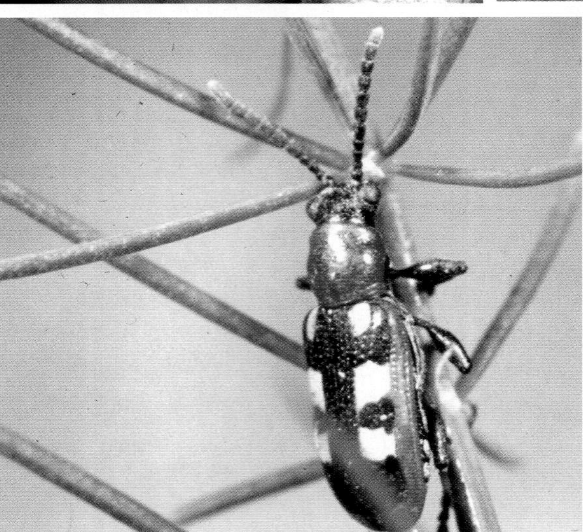

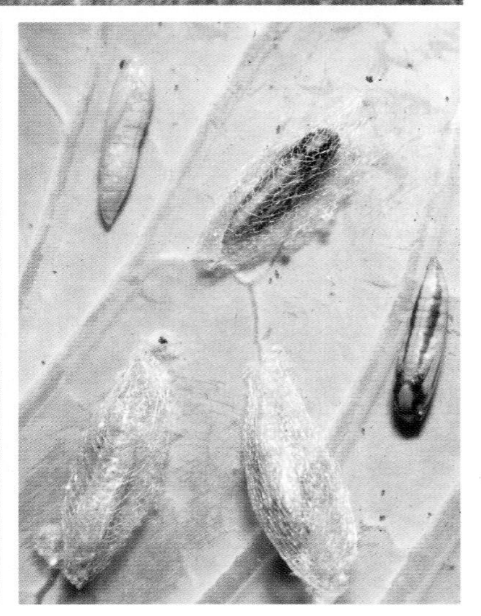

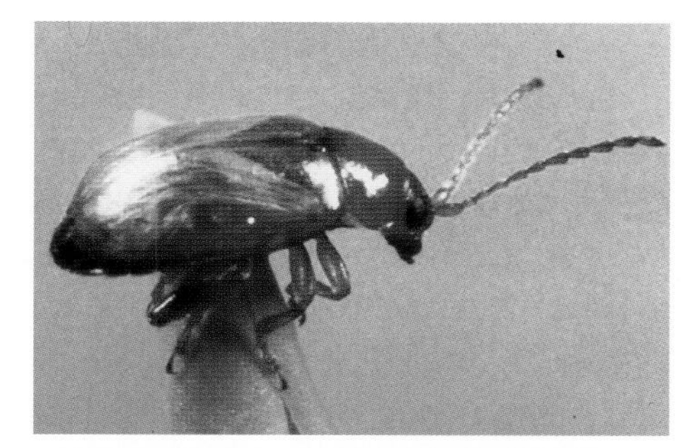

More pests, clockwise from below; Leafminer (*Ocym., Sat., Thuja*) - eriophyid mite damage (*Acon., All.c. Bell., Bov., Coccin., Mag.p., Nat.c., Ocym., Ricin., Salvia., Sil., Sul., Tromb., Thuja., Val., Vib.*) - the caterpillar of the diamondback moth and, above, the saddleback, (*Bombyx., Car., Coccin., Hyssop., Men., Nat.c., Ocym., Ricin., Salvia., Samb., Sat., Sil., Staphyl., Sul., Syrph., Tanac., Teuc., Thuja., Val., Vib.*) - mango seed weevil (*All.c., Aran., Ferr.s., Hyssop., Nat.c., Ocym., Sat., Staphylinida., Thuja.*) and the flea beetle (*Hys.*)

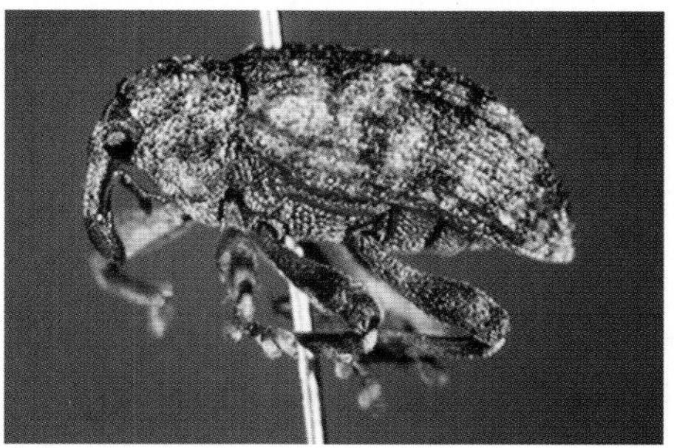

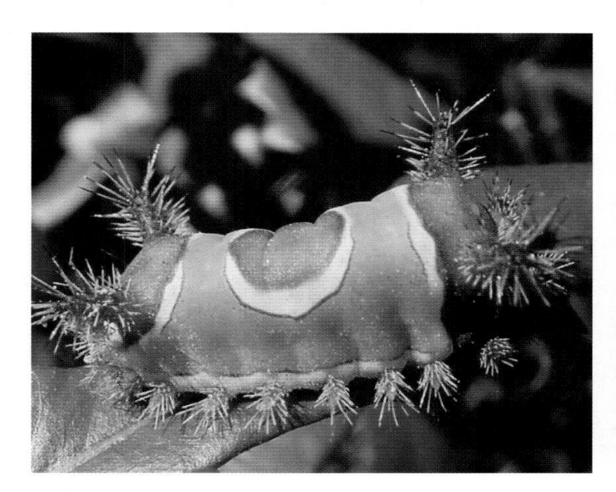

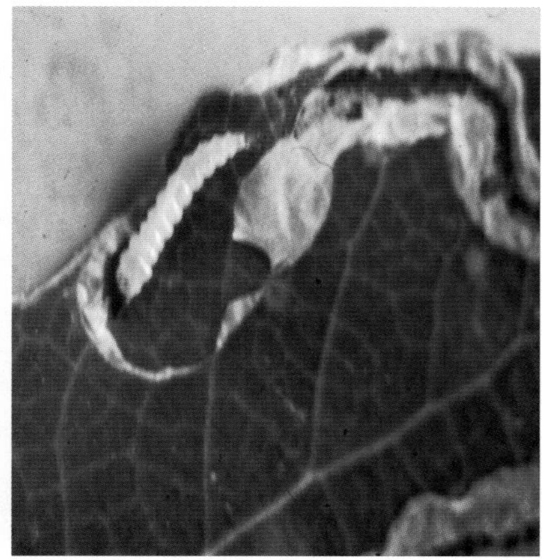

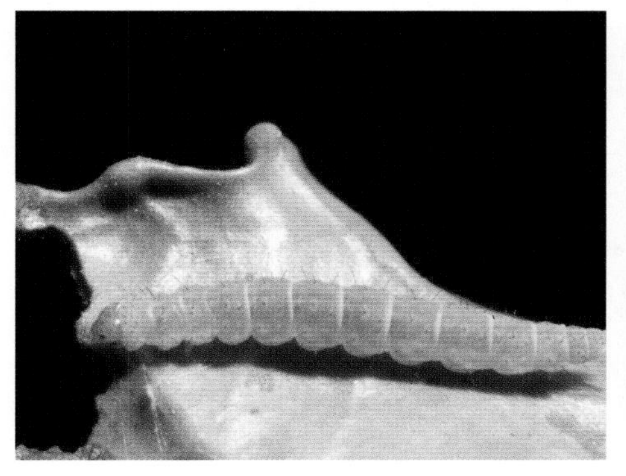

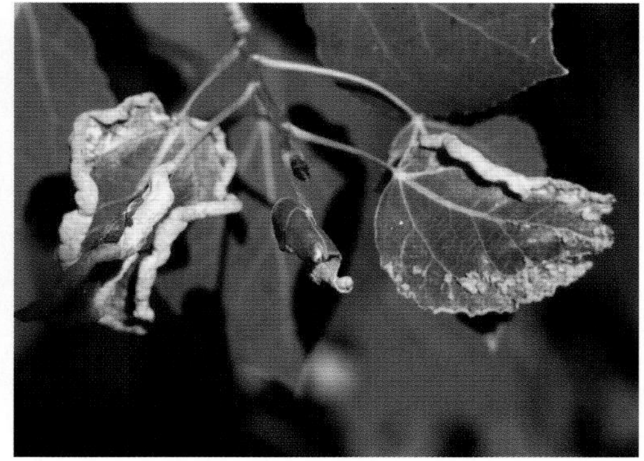

I am particularly keen that people feel welcome to join in with this work. Some aspects will, no doubt, remain open only to the well-funded and equipped experts - and such focused scrutiny is welcome. But everyone - gardeners, students, allotment holders, pensioners, gardening club members, small holders, schools, farmers, vintners, YOU - anyone with access to a patch of soil can try these non-toxic interventions. Then experiences can be collated to broaden the range of applications, to improve inaccurate assertions, and to deepen the confidence with successful remedies. After all this is how the homoeopathic work has developed with animals and humans.

We benefit from the technology to communicate and analyse data in ways that were not available to Hahnemann and the thousands of collaborators who have built the human materia medica over two hundred years. A site enquiring into the enigmas of biodynamic agriculture has been primed with the information in this materia medica. **http://www.considera.org** awaits your input. Those preferring more traditional methods are invited to submit their experiences to the publisher whose address is on the first page of this book.

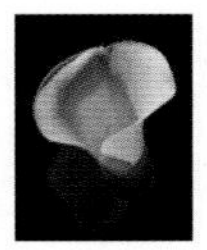

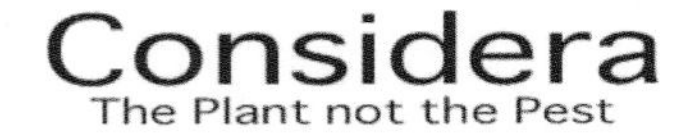

Considera
Planting by the Stars
Peppers
Preparations +
Introduction
Pioneers
Materia Medica
Repertory
Considera Ltd
Trees
Animals
Resources
Forum
Site Map
Contact

Materia Medica Agricultura

A *materia medica* is a catalogue of the sphere of influence of a remedy.

Here you can:-

- **Search** the existing materia medica
- **Add your own experiences** of the formulations to the materia medica
- If you are certain it doesn't already exist on this site, **add a remedy** to the materia medica. (Once you have done this you can add your experiences.)

"How to use the materia medica agricultura and its repertory". pdf 200 Kb download.

Please read if in **any** doubt, especially if you are making changes to the structure or content of the repertory.

| **Home** |

(Photographic credits on page 180)

(Salicylic Acid - continued from page 131)

The leaves of turnips and swedes show a clearing of the veins, coarse mottle, and dark green ring pattern. On stocks, plants can be stunted with distorted leaves, wrinkled and mottled with a lighter colour. Flowers are streaked with white or pale colours. These viruses are mainly spread by aphids. Cruciferous vegetables, annual flowers and weeds like shepherds purse, field cress, wild turnip, mustard and charlock are most affected by mosaic virus. The latter may be eradicated by *Natrum salicylicum*, *Salicylic acid* or *Lac* preparations.

RELATIONS
Compare: *Natrum salicylicum, Lac acid.*

Salvia Officinalis

Sage. NO *Labiatae*. Tincture of fresh leaves and blossom tips.

CLINICAL
Vine and *Brassicaceae* pests; mites, moths, aphids, cabbage fly. Other vine crops such as melon, cucumber, squash etc. Carrot fly. Weed control.

GENERAL
Salvia is another remedy from the order of *Labiatae*, and is equally effective as the other species. Because its range is limited to the vines and brassicas, we need to develop a remedy from the different species mixed together at mother tincture stage. This would produce a plant pest remedy of wide range - a plant/pest polychrest.

Because many remedies antidote each other in the potencies, complex prescribing is folly. Yet before potentisation, in the crude form, these plants do not antidote and as such can be made in a special tincture that comprises all the pest remedies of this order.

To this end, equal parts (in both weight and volume) of each plant are put together to produce the mother tincture, from which the potencies are produced. Provings will be conducted with these potencies on all types of plants and a diverse range of pests It will receive clinical tests.

Muller and Haines (1964) of the University of California Santa Barbara, observed that the dew gathered from Salvia contains a germination inhibitor. In potency it can be used in weed control.

Caution: do not apply on young plants.

Sambucus Nigra

Elder. NO *Caprifoliaceae*. Tincture of fresh leaves and flowers.

CLINICAL
General insect repellent, particularly against caterpillar. Bud worm, armyworm. Saw flies. Diamondback moth. Web worm, cut worm. Potato moth. Cluster caterpillar. Spitfire. Fly strike and rot in sheep. Oedematous swellings. Halo spot. Aphids.

GENERAL
Grows in hedges in moist places. When bruised, the leaves of the elder have an unpleasant odour which is offensive to most insects, and a decoction of these leaves is sometimes used by gardeners to keep caterpillars from delicate plants. It was the favourite medicinal plant of Hippocrates. The active ingredient in the crude is hydrocyanic acid. *Sambucus* was confirmed in the field after its description in the companion plant manuals. (Philbrick and Gregg, 1966.)

If sheep with rot can get at the bark and young leaves they will soon cure themselves. (Green, quoted by Clarke.) Millspaugh says that a decoction or ointment of flowers and leaves was applied to large wounds "to prevent deleterious effects from flies." (Millspaugh, 1892.) There is a relationship with *Valerian* and *Viburnum* on account of an identical acid present in the plants.

Oedematous swellings, especially in twigs, stems, and leaves. The capillaries do not give passage to sap, and waterlogging results in these places. The plant can take up carbon dioxide but cannot release oxygen. Evaporation is increased during the day, but ceases entirely at night.

RELATIONS
Compare: *Bombyx*, *Valerian*, *Viburnum*.

Satureia Hortensis

Savory. NO *Labiatae*. Tincture of the whole plant.

CLINICAL
Diseases and pests of beans. Mexican bean beetle, blossom thrips, bean fly, pod borer, angular leaf spot, anthracnose, bacterial brown spot, halo blight, leaf roll, rust, wilt. General insect repellent.

GENERAL
Savory is regarded as less effective than basil, although we have not been able to verify this. In its function as a companion plant it is, indeed, less effective than basil, but as the process of potentisation brings out increased medicinal power, the homoeopathic preparation does not have the disadvantage found in the companion plant. The recommendations of companion planting books - to go over the beans regularly, wiping off eggs and larvae of the Mexican bean beetle - are not necessary, when using the potency, thus saving many man-hours of labour.

From tests it has been proven to be equally effective for all pests and diseases in beans.

RELATIONS
As a prophylactic *Salicylic acid* can be used.
Compare *Natrum salicylicum, Salicylic acid*.

Secale Cornutum

Spurred rye. *Claviceps purpurea*. Ergot of rye. NO Fungi.

CLINICAL
Ergot, in all grains and grasses.

GENERAL
A black horn-like spur, into which the grains of rye are changed by the fungus *Claviceps purpurea*. Rye and other cereals such as grasses, are apt to be affected with ergot disease when grown on damp, ill-drained paddocks, which are waterlogged.

If breeding cattle are grazed on pastures where infected grasses grow, or are fed infected hay or straw, they are liable to drop their calves. This is a possible cause for brucellosis. The relation between ergot and brucellosis is not firmly established, but because the symptoms are so similar the correlation should be close. Secale generally miscarries at the seventh month and brucellosis does not occur before the seventh month, so it is tempting to make the link. (Allen, T. F., Hering, C., 1990.)

Brucellosis is very hard to eradicate by conventional means. The stables are usually treated with flame-throwers, and all cattle in the herd are generally slaughtered, yet the disease seems to take hold with equal vigour. A dose of *Secale* 30x given to cattle usually eradicates the disease whether caused by ergot or brucellosis, as my practice in India has proven time and time again. It is, however, advisable to treat the paddock with a 6x potency and remove all grain and straw that is suspected of infection from the feed stock. After spraying, it can be safely composted.

Because ergot affects all grains as well as grasses, *Secale* will cover all ergot species generically, given the fact that the properties of all grasses and grains in the materia medica do not differ very much, except in concomitants and modalities: compare Boericke's Materia Medica - alfalfa (*Medicago sativa*), stargrass (*Aletris farinosa*), sweet vernal grass (*Anoxanthum*), oats (*Avena Sativa*), buckwheat (*Fagopyrum*), goose grass (*Galium aparine*), knotgrass (*Polygonum aviculare*), and corn (*Stigmata maydis*).

All have disturbances in the generative sphere in a more or less pronounced degree, corresponding to the flowering and fruiting stage in plants. The symptoms listed below are <u>not</u> due to ergot.

Medicago: thirst, phosphate problems, flowers and fruits.
Aletris: flowers and fruits small or absent.
Avena: flowers and fruits disturbed, small or absent grains.
Fagopyrum: flowers and fruits disturbed, small or absent grains.
Galium: flowering affected.
Polygonum: thirst, flowers and fruits affected.
Stigmata maydis: flowers and fruits affected.

From these obvious similarities, it follows that *Secale* must have similar symptoms, which is further confirmed by the descriptions found in the materia medica. Another grain, *darnel*, is frequently infected with ergot, and many epidemics of miscarriage are due to this grain. It has had an evil reputation since ancient times and its name, means 'stupefied'. Mr. A. S. Wilson, in transactions of the Edinburgh Botanical society for 1874, declared that the poisonous properties of this grass are due to ergot which so commonly infects it. Note also that the cases of poisoning have been more frequently observed in low wet districts, and during the wet season. (Wilson, 1874; quoted by Clarke.)

APPEARANCE
Purple-black, horn-like ergots, replacing one or more seeds in the head. The ergots are larger than the grain. The first sign of infection is during flowering when yellowish droplets of sugary slime are produced.

Ergots survive in the soil for up to one year, producing spores which infect open wheat and other grain and grass florets. Infection is favoured by cool wet weather during flowering. Spores are spread by rain splash or insects attracted to the sugar. Ergots affect open pollinated species more than others. This is the main reason why most grain and grass species are affected. Hybrids are more often affected than other varieties, and oats and barley less.

Ergot is rare in Australia. Conventional control is not available. The best advise given by the grain board is to sow clean seed, allow one year fallow, or grow a different crop. Mowing or spraying a grass pasture to prevent flowering reduces ergot formation but with spraying it has the disadvantage of grass contaminated with herbicides.

Use of *Secale,* in practise in India, proved to be of excellent value in the control of brucellosis in cattle and the subsequent effects in humans. At the same time the pastures were treated to eradicate ergot in the grains and grasses.

NOTE
Secale cereale in two successive crops eradicates couch grass, chick weed and most other weeds.

Silicea

Pure flint. Silica terra. Silex. *Silicon dioxide*. SiO_2. Trituration of pure precipitated silica. Remedy sometimes also known as Silicia and Silica.

CLINICAL
Die back. Premature flowering, herbicide, germination aid, general tonic, transplant shock, soil remedy, weak straggly plants, puny growth, bark and sheath diseases, chlorosis, aphids, bud worm, citrus mite, dried fruit beetle.

GENERAL:
Outside homoeopathy, flint as a remedy for internal use is unknown. Hahnemann introduced it into medicine. Through his method of attenuating insoluble substances, its medicinal powers have been liberated and revealed. A large proportion of the Earth's crust is composed of silica. Sea sand (*Silica marina*) is mostly composed of it. Silica is taken up by plants and is deposited on the interior of the stems as well as forming the sheath or bark that holds the plant upright. "Want of grit" is the leading indication for *Silicea*.

Silica type plants grow in sandy soils and there one will find few problems. It is plants that do not belong in those soils who experience problems.

Silicic acid is a constituent of the cells of the connective tissue. The epidermis forms the protective sheath around the cambium where silica gives strength to the long molecules of the fibre. *Silicea* will cripple bark in healthy trees causing death. The suppuration it can set up is sufficient to destroy a plant or tree. Its indication in dieback has been confirmed in practice with remarkable results. A sapling with dieback, which had only one quarter of the bark left, which was loose and drying out, was given one dose of *Silicea* 6x and the next day, the bark was reattached to the cambium, and after one week, the top branches were growing new shoots and leaves.

Silicea is one of the key remedies in agricultural homoeopathy, as our tests have so far confirmed.

If one understands *Silicea* and its extensive range of action, one will not meet with many difficulties elsewhere. What *Natrum muriaticum* is for the law of potency, is what *Silicea* is for plants. No other remedy has a deeper action on the life of plants, and no other remedy has so wide a spectrum. It is the true polychrest of agriculture, much more so than any other nutrient. Without silica, no plant can stand upright. It acts on every cell and tissue of the whole plant, giving grit and strength, regulating all cellular processes including reproduction.

Silicic acid is the most extensive element of the earth's crust or the lithosphere. In plants, silicic acid forms the supportive substance. It is abundant in algae, equisetum, polygonum and the grasses (Graminae). In birds, the ashes of the feathers have a particularly high content.

Silica is not restricted to a supportive function in plants. As a hydrophile colloid, it can retain many times its own weight of water. Plants growing on stony or arid soils are able to create a considerable water reserve due to this water retentive property. The increased absorption on silica-rich soils in desert biomes such as found extensively in Australia, proves its capacity to delay drying out. One dose of *Silicea* is usually sufficient to help generate the seeds of perennials and biennials so that they can lead healthy lives from the moment they are sown.

Silica is an element of the moon, that is it has great formative powers. Silica, as a building block, rivals carbon in rank of importance to plant life and in the production of protective tissues.

Another feature of *Silicea* is its capacity to set up premature flowering. This opens up possibilities as a herbicide, as it prevents seed formation in annual weeds. Here it must be used twice in 10 days (and more). To prevent weeds coming up or causing problems in broad-acre, spray *Silicea* twice or more in 10 days, to prevent seed forming, then sow the desired crop with the last application.

A third indication is as an aid to germination. Here it must be given only once at planting time. The plant will grow strong roots and firm shoots and leaves. A further application is as a tonic for weak plants that are puny.

Given after flowering, *Silicea* will help fruit setting. All these applications have been tested in the field whereby many of the features came as unanticipated reactions. They confirm the findings of Rudolf Steiner and have given a few more indications. They went far beyond expectations and showed that *Silicea* ranks as one of the most important remedies with which tests have been conducted.

From the materia medica we can learn some of the specific uses of *Silicea*. It looks possible to attempt to regain the desert with less heartache and speculation with the help of *Silicea* and *Calcarea, Equisetum* and *Polygonum.* Hahnemann gave us the hint that the environment in which the patient lives must be given high priority. A desert is mainly sand, especially so in Australia. The earlier statement of Hering about the previous medicinal power with the strongest influence, alluded to the consequent treatment.

Homoeopathy has many other uses that can improve the quality of life, or even of the products that we make. The idea is a lot less fanciful than it may first appear. On sandy soils *Silicea* works wonders in spite of a harsh environment (or even thanks to such circumstances). *Silicea* can make plants thrive. It can be used in soils where all appears normal yet puny plants persist, and on any plant at sowing time. It is good as protection against mildew and mould, for weak cells, exhaustion, fruit setting, striking, transplanting, green manure provision, all bark diseases and dieback. In short, like no other remedy, *Silicea* and silica preparations have an effect on every stage of a plant's life, are universally applicable at any stage, have a profound action, with long duration, from one single application.

Silicea is a soil remedy of prime order. It is the antidote to *Manganum* in manganese toxicity. In sandy soils it changes the ionisation of the particles from water repellent to water absorbent. The negative effects of sandy soils are counteracted, and plants immediately begin to thrive. It is from tests with this form of application that the idea of a germination aid was conceived, and was visible in the germination of grass.

Silica preparations must be used with caution because, just as *Silicea* can help green a desert, it can as quickly create one with devastating effects. *Silicea* is one of the great powers in nature, capable of destruction as well as healing depending on the skill of the practitioner.

Silicea gave excellent results at Port Bouvard Bowling Club, where patches of bare ground were covered in turf in less than two weeks. 10 x 4 m patches were quickly covered with strong grass, which has little or no problem with the ever present fairy ring spot. We do not hesitate to use it when circumstances demand it.

To date, bowling greens are greener, dollar dead spot is cured, timber grass is taller and stronger, plants stay healthier and timber is harder and denser, thus more termite free. Trees are less prone to dieback, dieback is cured, plants are resistant to pests and diseases, and firmer, larger fruits are produced - all thanks to *Silicea*.

APPEARANCE
Chlorotic, weak, stunted plants that fail to thrive. Failure to regrow after transplants - the plant is green but does not take. Slimy roots. Need for nutrients, but inability to assimilate. Brittle stems and twigs breaking under strain. Weakness in the generative sphere; small puny flowers, little or no pollen, immature stamen, fruits refuse to mature, and fall before maturity. Hardness of leaves and bark, leather-leaf, red spots, ulcerating wounds from pruning, storm or mechanical damage. Burrowing under bark galls, tree cancers.

FLOWERS AND FRUITS
Weakness in generative sphere, immature flowers and fruits, no seed forming, bud worm.

WATER NEEDS
Need more nutrients than water.

NOTE
Silicea has many uses, however, selection of *Silicea* must follow given criteria and must be used with caution.

RELATIONS
Compare: *Lapis albus.*
Antidote to: *Manganum.*
Complementary: *Calcarea.*

Sulphur

Brimstone. S. Sublimated sulphur. Trituration of flowers of sulphur. A saturated solution in absolute alcohol constitutes the mother tincture.

CLINICAL
Fruit-piercing moth, dried fruit beetle, fruit fly, fruit spotting bug, droopy plants, worse after rain. Capillary congestion. Plants emaciated, straggly, thin, weak. Ailments from raw, cutting winds. Worse from warmth, sun, rain, cold damp weather. Root nematode, root gall, crown gall, spots, rust, blotch blight, mildew, moulds, rots, both dry and slimy. Leather leaf, blister mites, two-spotted mites.

GENERAL
Sulphur is an elementary substance, occurring in nature as a brittle crystalline solid, burning in the air with a blue flame, being oxidised to sulphur dioxide. The reputation of *Sulphur* as a remedy is perhaps as old as medicine itself. As early as 2000 years ago, says Hahnemann, "*Sulphur* had been used as the most powerful specific agent against the itch". (Hahnemann, 1834.)

The domestic use of *Sulphur* as a spring medicine is based on its antipsoric properties. It is this property of *Sulphur*, to divert to the surface constitutional irritants, which renders it the chief of Hahnemann's antipsorics. It is a powerful antiseptic, in no way limited to psora. Cooper states that workers in sulphur mines, though in malarial districts, remain immune from intermittent fevers.

In plants the capillary system is disturbed so as to cause irregular distribution of circulation: congestion, inflammation in rusts and blotches, redness, runs through the remedy. Sluggish circulation. Defective assimilation, emaciation, thin straggly plants that get plenty of nutrients. Dried up plants which are yellowish and flabby. Photosynthesis is greatly impaired and disturbed. Worse in the heat of summer, worse at night, periodicity of 12 hours.

A dose of crude Sulphur improves the qualities for milling and baking in wheat when given shortly before the harvest. (Randall, 1990.)

Sulphur gets fixed by excess levels of nitrogen or ammonia. It is through the remedies with either ammonia or nitrogen in their composition that these effects can be antidoted. *Kali nitricum* can only be used in this respect when there is also a potassium imbalance. (Spencer et al. 1977.)

Sulphur is the chronic of *Aconite* in rusts and where *Aconite* fails to cure, *Sulphur* will rapidly cure.

Sulphur acts on all aspects of photosynthesis from the leaves to the storage of protein. It has an alternation between problems with photosynthesis and rust eruption. The plant is always worse after rain. Congestion of single parts; roots, stems, leaves or flowers.

In 1966, Wannamaker treated seedlings with dilutions of Sulphur from 12x to 20m, using controls. The weight and dimensions of the seedlings plus their contents of sodium, potassium, calcium and magnesium, were affected in a significant fashion. (Wannamaker, 1966.)

Sulphur does not give a response as a fertiliser component in plants, unless accompanied by phosphorus, calcium or sodium. (See *Calcarea sulphurica*, *Natrum sulphuricum*.) A sulphur deficiency is notable when the level of sulphur is lower than 300 ppm. Sulphur of deficient plants had levels of SO_4 of 120 - 220 ppm. The amount of dry matter is the standard measurement in most tests, for either toxicity or deficiency. Sulphur deficiencies in the field can only be determined by reduced or limited growth. (Mason et al. 1974.)

Sulphur needs to be processed in the soil, as plants only take up the sulphate. Thus calcium sulphate, or sodium sulphate are some of the forms in which it can be applied. *Calcarea sulphuricum* on alkaline and acid soils can help the plant recover in a short time. On salt affected areas *Natrum sulphuricum* will be indicated. In sandy soils, little sulphate is available due to both retention problems and difficulties with adsorption. Leaching is the main problem on sandy soils, which can be reduced through the buildup of organic content in the soil.

Chlorosis and retardation of growth and maturity are the main symptoms in cereals. Nitrogen is of importance as an inimical to sulphur. The plant becomes entirely yellow while the stems redden. Nitrogen has similar symptoms but affects the older leaves first. All cereal crops are highly susceptible to sulphur deficiency. (Yeates, 1978.)

Sulphur is a constituent of amino acids and so is essential in the formation of proteins. Sulphur is partially mobile in plants, hence the symptoms are visible in both the young and the older leaves.

Ailments from heavy metal poisoning, regardless of the metal; cobalt, lead, arsenic, zinc, cadmium. *Sulphur* is frequently needed where acute diseases do not clear up completely.

APPEARANCE
The roots are dry or slimy, with blisters or vesicles. Epidermis comes off the roots as in root nematode, root gall, crown gall. Plants very thirsty. Great need for nutrients with impaired assimilation. Photosynthesis is impaired, lack of oxygen carriers and subsequent congestion of the leaves. Violent capillary congestion, fluids stagnate, sugars not produced, no nitrogen uptake from the atmosphere. Premature flowering, before season, defective pollination. Sterility, no fruit, seed or grains produced.

Sulphur is the greatest general remedy for eruptions. Rust, blotch, blight, mildew, moulds and stripe. Herbicide damage. Rots, both dry and slimy.

Leather leaf. Spots with buff centres surrounded by a diffuse red brown aura are characteristic. As the disease progresses, whole leaves may be covered. The leaves become stiff, rolled and have a leathery appearance. The disease is most severe in high rainfall areas such as the south east of South Australia and Western districts of Victoria. Dry spells will curb the disease spread.

Visual symptoms of sulphur deficiency may vary widely throughout the same genus of plants provided the subspecies are different. At the 2-4 leaf stage, there may be pinkish discolouration on the leaf mid ribs or parallel veins. This is usually browner on nitrogen-deficient plants and there is no discolouration on stems and cotyledons as in nitrogen deficiency. Sometimes the leaves curl inwards. Purpling then increases in the interveinal areas. The leaves that newly develop are narrower than normal. The flowers are pale. The purpling spreads to the stem, petioles and mid ribs. Sometimes the pink is deep shade, especially on the underside of the leaves. New leaves are poorly developed while older leaves turn orange before dying.

Sulphur-based herbicides such as Sulfonylurea can reduce the uptake of copper. (Robson and Snowball, 1990, McCay and Robson, 1992, Black and Wilhelm, 1991.)

RELATIONS
Inimical to: *Cuprum, Ammonium, Molybdenum, Nitricum acidum.*
Complementary: *Aconite.*
Follows well: *Aconite.*
Antidote to: *Calcarea, Cobalt, Cuprum, Cadmium, Plumbum, Arsenicum album, Mercurius.*
Antidoted by: *Zinc.*

Tanacetum Vulgare

Tansy. NO *Compositae*. Tincture of whole flowering plant.

CLINICAL
Flies, worms of any type, Japanese beetles, ants, moths, fleas. Rabies. Nematodes. Peach is most affected by *Tanacetum*. Premature fruit drop.

GENERAL
Grows on high ground and pastures. Tanacetum oil is, according to Hale (quoted by Clarke), identical with Santonin, thus explaining the vermifugal action of *Tanacetum*. Besides this, Peyraud (quoted by Clarke) has used tansy as a substitute for vaccinations against rabies. In Russia it is used as a substitute for hops in beer. It has a camphorous odour. Worm expellant in cattle and sheep.

From herbals (Grieve, 1931, Hylton, 1974, and others), it has been found that as a plant it repels flies, Japanese beetles and ants.

In potency it is taken up by the plant and this confers immunity against some pests. It is especially useful to keep ants away from plants infested with aphids, as ladybird larvae can not feed as easily on aphids protected by ants.

Teucrium Marum

Cat thyme. *Marum verum*. NO *Labiatae*. Tincture of whole fresh plant.

CLINICAL
Thread worm. Cabbage root fly. Moths. Nematodes. Mastitis in cows. Flowering and fruit setting problems.

GENERAL
There exists no other remedy that meets cases of nematodes better than *Teucrium*. Nematodes inhibit plant growth and impede respiration, especially the root knot nematode (Meloidogyne spp.). In potato tubers the whole of the tuber becomes lumpy. Some other remedies like *Calendula* also can be used for nematode control.

From the symptoms listed in the Materia Medica, references can be drawn in regard to nutrient levels - both nematode and *Teucrium* symptoms are identical.

In companion planting the species of *Teucrium* are not as effective as *Ruta* but in potency, do confer immunity to pests. All species of thyme have this capacity, the *Thymus* varieties equally so.

From different herbals (Grieve, 1931, Hylton, 1974) and companion plant books (Hemphill, 1990, Philbrick and Gregg, 1966) it can be learned that dried thyme repels moths in the wardrobe.

Many tests are still to be conducted to establish the full range of *Teucrium* preparations.

RELATIONS
Compare: *Mentha*.

Thuja

Yellow cedar. Thuja occidentalis. *Arbor vitae*. Tree of life. NO *Coniferae*. Tincture of fresh green twigs.

CLINICAL
Pests in general, mites, hawk moth, scale, blister mite, rust mite. Pests in *Cucurbitae*. Cancer in trees. Galls. Farcy and grease in horses. Fungus gall.

GENERAL
Grows upon the rocky banks of rivers, low swampy spots. The volatile oil is used in the West Indies as a powerful insecticide.

Teste mentions in his Materia Medica that thuja wood does not decay. He also disagrees with Hahnemann's idea of a signature, regarding the "resinous callosities of the stems and leaves of thuja might have seemed an indication that the plant is a specific for sycosis and warts". (Teste, 1974.)

Sycosis is according to Hahnemann the constitutional disease resulting from constitutional (i.e. hereditary) gonorrhoea. The characteristic manifestations are warts, either dry or soft, cancers and cauliflower excrescences.

From the provings it appears that Hahnemann was right and this is corroborated by Kent. Hering says that it acts on the fluids causing: ". . . dissolution of the fluids, which become acrid. It disturbs the digestion." In the vegetable sphere: "A surplus of producing life; nearly unlimited proliferation of pathological vegetation, condylomata warty, sycotic excresences, spongy tumours. All morbid manifestations are excessive, but appear quietly, so that their beginning is scarcely known. "(Hering, 1990.)

Through analogous diagnosis, this can easily be related to galls, either hard or soft, or soft cankerous growth on trees. A good example is the fungus gall of wattles (*Uromycladeum* spp.).

Many borers can be treated with *Thuja*, as it is a remedy that can neutralise "animal poisons" such as vaccination and its negative effects in humans. Thus many insects that attack plants and trees will respond to this remedy especially if disease is the result of pest attack, like barley yellow dwarf virus, mosaic virus and other viral and bacterial disease.

Much testing has to be done to confirm this, although analogy also here is the leading feature for its indications. Giving *Thuja* "internally", i.e. watering the roots, so it can be taken up, produces more striking effects than spraying, as was found in some of the tests.

Trombidium

Trombidium muscae domesticae. NO Arachidnae. Tincture of the insect.

CLINICAL
Carriers: housefly, stable fly, blow fly. Worse manuring, watering, cold rainy weather. Red spider mite.

GENERAL
Trombidium is a parasite found on the common housefly. It is bright red and nearly circular. The alcoholic tincture, a brilliant orange in colour, was prepared from around a hundred specimens collected in Frankfort Philadelphia, in September 1864. Although Clarke presents this as a "parasite of the house fly", modern research suggests it is a species of *Tarsonemus* mite, which, considering its orange red colour, is the red spider mite which swarms by attaching itself to the fly (Hussey, 1981). Thus it falls in the Order of *Arachidnae.*

The mite breeds in compost and manure, feeds on mycelium of different species of fungi found in manures mixed with straw. It also attacks the mycelium of developing spores of edible mushrooms and is a serious pest among mushroom growers worldwide.

The grand keynote of *Trombidium* is worse from nutrients and watering. Any pest or disease that gets worse from the application of fertiliser or water will improve under *Trombidium*. Blotches and patches, more prevalent on hairy leaves.

Roots may have mould and poor assimilation of nutrients. The capillaries seem congested. Leaves, especially in hairy species, may show spots. The respiration, photosynthesis, and evaporation are all disturbed. From extensive tests by the USDA it has been observed that plants with excess potassium and phosphorus are more prone to aphid and mite attack, while pest numbers increase more rapidly on over-fed plants.

RELATIONS
Compare: *Bovista*.

Urea

Carbamide. The chief solid substance in the urine of mammals (white crystals). $CO(NH_2)_2$. Trituration or solution.

CLINICAL
Problems with photosynthesis, capillary system and leaves (chlorosis).

GENERAL
Urea has been used in agriculture as a fertiliser. Without it, plants are chlorotic with concomitant photosynthesis problems and sluggish circulation in the capillary system, which results in engorgement and puffiness. Cooper mentions that a celebrated breeder of cattle and horses succeeded in getting his animals skin into an astonishing condition of fineness by giving his animals a tablespoon of old human urine with each meal.

Urine has been used as an insecticide since ancient times, probably due to its level of ammonia, producing nitrogen in the soil. It had a double function.

RELATIONS
Compare: A*mmonium, Nitricum acidum, Kali Nitricum.*
Antidote to: *Molybdenum.*
Complementary: *Molybdenum.*

Ustilago

Corn smut. NO Fungi. Trituration.

CLINICAL
Smut, flag smut, bunt, loose smut, head scab. Found on oats, sorghum, wheat, barley, triticale and corn.

GENERAL
Like *Secale*, with which it should be compared, *Ustilago* affects animals that feed on grains affected with smut in a similar manner; they miscarry. Roullin remarks that, "sheep lose their wool, mules cast their hoofs, and chickens lay eggs without shells" (quoted by Clarke).

Like *Secale*, *Ustilago* has an affinity for the generative sphere. Clarke mentions a case of a female dog losing five foetuses at the fifth week of gestation, and all hair on her body whilst her nails were loose. In plants, the bark will loosen, and it may well prove to be another remedy like *Silicea*, which arrests dieback.

Flag smut. (*Urocystis tritici*)
Long grey raised streaks on the leaves, shafts and stems. Heads badly damaged. These streaks break through, showing masses of grey black spores which are spread on clothes, animals and insects. Affected leaves are twisted and split lengthwise. Stunted plants give early warning, although spotting them is not always easy. Tillers will perpetuate the damage on future crops. Spores are wind borne and survive for several years. Early sowing during warm weather favours and promotes infection.

WATER NEEDS
Likes evening watering. Appears wilted in the morning.

Bunt. (*Neovossia indica - Tilletia indica*)
Bunt is difficult to spot, but at maturity smutted heads can be seen, grey brown bunts replacing the grain, the balls forcing the glumes apart. Infected plants are shorter and stay green longer, taking more time to mature. The balls break and release spores during harvest. Fishy odour. Cool and moist conditions favour infection at planting time. The fungus grows through the plant affecting only the head. Infection is less likely in warmer temperatures. Even resistant varieties may become affected, especially when blight is severe. Spores remain dormant for up to several years.

WATER NEEDS
Normal.

Head scab. (*Fusarium* spp)
Head scab is classified under the action of smuts and covered by *Ustilago*. Cattle do not like this stock and when fed with head scab infected grains will miscarry, become

infertile, develop haemorrhage of the intestinal canal and refuse food. There is no conventional chemical control available for smuts.

Premature bleaching of a section or all of a head. Pink and orange fungal strands appear over the head. Infected areas are most often sterile. Seeds are shrivelled and have a pinkish colour. Head scab survives in the soil, on cereal residue and grass. The spores are spread by rain splash. Moist conditions and warm to hot weather are most favourable to this fungus.

WATER NEEDS
Normal.

Loose smut. (*Ustilago nuda* spp tritici)
When the heads emerge, a mass of dark brown powdery spores can be seen. Initially, the spores are held in a thin membrane which soon breaks. All that remains of the head is a bare stalk and some drift. Spores are wind borne and affect other wheat and barley crops. Moist, warm conditions favour infection. Infected grain is not visibly different from healthy grain until the heads emerge.

WATER NEEDS
Normal.

Valeriana

Valerian. *Valeriana officinalis*. NO *Valerianacea*. Tincture of fresh root.

CLINICAL
Slimy mould, moulds in general, banana rust thrips. Nematodes.

GENERAL
Valerian is usually found off ditches and streams, thus its use for waterlogged soil. What *Sambucus* cured in the plant was waterlogging in leaves, and here the soil is waterlogged, giving rise to the associated problems. Valerian has a peculiar kind of smell that repels insects on man, plant and animal.

Roots have a whitish blistery appearance. The plant takes up nutrients well, but seems not to thrive. Protein content is low, photosynthesis impaired. Uptake of CO_2 is diminished due to clogging of the pores in the epidermis of the leaves. Evaporation is increased. The flowers come too early or poorly developed. *Valeriana* stimulates phosphorus activity. It attracts earth worms. It can be used on all plants.

The plant feels better in windy weather, rather than wind still. The leaves show rust patches, confluent rather than isolated, as from banana rust thrips. Alternatively, there may be moulds - shiny moulds in particular.

FLOWERS AND FRUITS
Flowers very early, with incomplete development. Banana rust thrips.

Banana rust thrips (*Chaetanaphothrips signipennis*:) adults, yellow in colour, 1.5mm long nymph, 1mm and paler in colour. Feed between fruits and under leaves. Reddish areas develop on the plant, fruit damage more serious. Rough skin, dull grey, flecked with red. Later turning to red brown, skin splits, numerous from January to March. Look for them from October on pseudo-stems and bunches. In the Southern hemisphere, August to October, but look for them in April.

WATER NEEDS
High, due to high evaporation rate.

RELATIONS
Compare: *Bombyx, Sambucus, Viburnum.*

Viburnum Opulus

High cranberry bush. Cramp bark. Water elder. NO *Caprifoliaceae*. Tincture of fresh bark.

CLINICAL
General insect repellent.

GENERAL
Grows on river banks. In America, the wild species, says Hale, is called "cramp bark". The American Indians used it in spasmodic diseases. Viburnum smells like Valerian or *Elder* and has equal repellent qualities to the others. Hale tells us further that, in the generative sphere, it can prevent early dropping of fruit if applied at the first sign.

The roots look pale and the epidermis may be dry. Nutrients may not be taken up. CO_2 uptake is also defective, plant is low in protein or starch. As with *Sambucus* and *Valeriana*, *Viburnum* has profuse evaporation. The leaves do not release CO_2 at night. Photosynthesis and respiration are not up to par. The whole digestive system is severely affected whilst the capillary system appears inactive. The female parts of the flowers are affected resulting in early dropping of fruits. Timely application of *Viburnum* will help fruits to mature and ripen before they fall.

WATER NEEDS
Normal to higher need.

RELATIONS
Compare: *Bombyx, Sambucus, Valeriana.*

Zincum

Elemental zinc. Zn Trituration of the metal.

CLINICAL
Potato scab, apple and citrus scab, powdery scab, rhizoctonia scab, violet scab, turf and root nematodes.

GENERAL
Zinc belongs to the magnesium group of metals. It has long been known in the arts. Together with copper it is used in the manufacture of brass. Zinc poisons the brain and nerves in humans and animals. In plants the tissues are worn out faster than they can be replaced. The so-called 'scrapie' in sheep and mad cows disease are possibly due to zinc poisoning and can be treated successfully with *Zinc* preparations.

Zinc is essentially a trace element. It is essential to the auxins in cell division and multiplication and in the breakdown of carboxyl compounds, which in excess are toxic to plants. The visible symptoms show as pale green and yellow leaves. In severe cases they turn dark green. Older leaves are first affected and this may later extend to the younger leaves and shoots. The leaftip turns yellow and as the symptoms spread the tips may turn orange, then red, and finally grey and black. All stages of this colour change may be present in a single leaf.

Oat glumes are darkened and leaves will twist from the tip down. Oats are more susceptible than wheat and barley. Less than 12 ppm is considered deficient, 20 ppm is seen as normal. (Brennan, 1988.)

In wheat the symptoms are more severe in clouded weather and wet and cool soils. The signs start on the middle leaves and extend to the new growth. Along the midvein of fully emerged leaves a pale strip is visible, which later turns brown and becomes necrotic. Then the colour turns grey. Chlorosis is sometimes prominent. The leaves may look succulent i.e. waterlogged. Yellow mottled areas may surround the necrotic patches. The plants then show drooped leaves. (Brennan, 1986.)

Zinc deficiency in plants causes a yellowing of leaves in the same direction as the veins and begins close to the veins spreading over the leaves. It is different from chlorosis due to lack of iron, in that the yellow is more towards a tan colour, thus confusion of the remedy is eliminated. Zinc has a strong action on the generative sphere. It causes premature pollination and consequent diminished fruits. Capillary system is engorged in the leaves; veins stand out. The roots have vesicles, in potato scab, root knot nematodes. Plants are thirsty, leaves show chlorosis with impaired photosynthesis and capillary engorgement. In the flowers, premature pollination and consequent sterility.

Some sulphur-based herbicides will result in a lowering of the uptake of zinc in the plant. Zinc deficiency causes growth reduction in terminal limbs and a condition called 'little leaf'. The shoots have shorter internodes. Rosette appearance of shoot tips. Delay or failure to shoot, with leaf loss. Interveinal chlorosis with pointed leaves. Dieback of the limbs. Delayed flowering or complete absence of flowers. Tardy fruitdrop and failure to set fruit. (Shorter and Cripps, 1985.) Zinc deficiency can also result in stunting. Fleck symptoms of and on the upper leaves, which spreads into necrosis of the leaf. (Mason and Gartrell, undated.)

Common scab (*Streptomycin* scabies).
This disease, also known as 'potato scab', begins as small brown dots on the tubers. As the tuber grows, the dots increase in size and can cover most of the surface. Symptoms may vary from raised corky areas to deep pits. It is usually brought in by infected planting stock. It appears first on the leaves and shows spots of 3 mm in a different green. It occurs on limestone and alkaline soils and in dry seasons. Zinc deficiency promotes it. Affects potatoes, turnip, beetroot.

Apple scab (*Venturia* spp.).
This disease is also known as 'black spot'. They darken and become black, forming large patches. The fruits develop black spots which turn brown and corky. Young fruit becomes distorted with cracks. The spores are spread by rain splash. It develops in fallen leaves during winter. In spring, spores infect new growth through wind dispersion. In damp weather at around 15 degrees, wet leaves become infected. In some regions, infection time is broadcast so that spray programs can be accurately timed. Also here zinc plays an important role in both toxicity and deficiency.

Plants affected: Granny Smith, Delicious, Jonathan, Gravenstein. Pear scab is similar but cannot cross-infect apples and vice versa.

Root knot nematode (Meloidogyne spp.)
These nematodes seem to cause more problems in light soils and warm climates. They are 0.5 mm long, thin transparent bodies which cannot be seen with the naked eye. The males are in the soil, whilst the females are found in the roots. Eggs are deposited in the soil in a gelatinous mass or in the outer layers of the roots. Up to 2000 eggs are produced by the female. After hatching, the larvae enter young roots near the tip.

Their saliva causes super large cells, as in cancer, so that the root becomes bumpy. The roots then branch, and the nematodes attack the tip so that a knot is formed. Potato tubers will become bumpy as in common scab. These tubers cannot feed the plant above ground which appears slow-growing, stunted, wilting readily in hot weather. Leaves are paler green than normal. These nematodes spread through running water, tractor wheels, shoes, spades and ploughs, and infested plants.

RELATIONS
Antidoted by: *Sulphur, Zinc.*
Inimical: *Kali. Molybdenum.*
Antidote to: *Ferrum, Sulphur.*
Compare: Nematodes, *Calendula, Tanacetum vulgare.*

Repertory

Currently the materia medica is too small for comprehensive and effective diagnosis of all plant diseases. But, as has been done with the immense volume of information for humans, it makes sense to create a structured index even at this early stage. This is called a 'repertory'.

In order to find the remedy for a problematic situation, note the position of any 'presenting symptom' on the plant, for instance on the fruits, flowers, leaves, stem or roots. Note the type of symptom, that is, the damage in the form of blotches, spots, flecks, chlorosis, pest, either stationary, moving, larva, or other instar, and whether it has wings, etc.

Record any events in the plants' history which seem relevant such as an injury from which it has never really recovered.

Last but not least come the concomitants: what appears at the same time as the main symptoms, and modalities, that is if the plants are worse or better at any particular time of day, temperature, or weather pattern.

Remedies are shown in plain type, *in italics* and **in bold face**. The bold type remedies have been found to assist the relevant 'rubric' or symptom consistently, the italic ones often and the plain type ones occasionally.

All these single presenting symptoms can be looked up in the repertory and certain remedies are likely to feature several times. These are the remedies that should then be studied in the materia medica and the most appropriate remedy, or 'similimum', selected and administered.

The repertory follows the same tried and tested format as for humans. It is helpful to find as many symptoms as possible, especially those that are strange rare or peculiar. If some symptoms are particular to one remedy only, they are graded as most important and are the indicative symptoms or 'keynotes'. The more keynotes obtained, the easier it is to find the appropriate remedy.

Visible symptoms always take precedence over laboratory reports or microscopic evidence. This is because laboratory reports and other evidence may be hard to come by, or because the symptoms set in with great speed and time is of the utmost importance.

It would be appreciated if you would report inconsistencies, inaccuracies, or obvious incorrect information, so that future editions may be corrected. It is also appreciated when clear results are reported, so that this method can be updated and spread to more users in the future.

General

brittle; Calc.p.
discolouration**:**
  black: **Arn., Calend.**
  brown; Calc.p.
  blue: Arn., Calend., **Nat.sal., Sal.ac.**
  bluegreen: Arn., Calend., Nat.sal. Sal.ac. Zinc m.
  lightgreen: Arn., Calend.
  orange: **Acon., Amm.carb.**, Berb., Kali m.
  pink: Sul.
  purple: **Nat.sal.**, *Nit.ac.*, **Sal.ac.**, Sul.
  red: **Acon., Amm.carb., Bell.**, Berb., *Canth.*, **Carbo v.**, Cham. Sul.
  yellow: **Acon., Amm.carb.,** Arn., **Bell.** Berb., *Canth.*, Kali m., Sul.
  white; Sul.
congestion:
  of single parts: Sul.
deformed**:**
  engorged: Arn., Calc., Calend.
  shrivelled: Equis., Sil.
  with:
    bacterial disease: Ferr.m., **Nat.sal., Sal.ac**.
    capillary paralysis: Acon., Arn. Ferr.m., Ferr.p.
    fungal disease: **Acon., Amm carb., Bell.** Berb., *Canth*., **Equis**., Phos., **Sil.**
    nematodes: *Calend*., Carbo v., Nast., **Tanac**., **Teuc.**, Val.
    pest activity: Acon., All.c., Amm.c., Aran., Bell., **Bombyx**., Car., **Coccin**. **Chrysop**., Hyssop. Kali c., Men., Nast., **Nat.sal**., Nat.sul., Ocym., Ricin., **Ruta**., **Sal.ac**., Salvia., Samb., Sat., Sil., **Staphyl., Syrph.**, Tanac., **Teuc.**, Thuja.
epidermis:
  cracks; Calc.p.
  dry: Berb., Bov., Equis., Sil.. Sul., Vib.
  erruptions; Sul.
  engorged; **Arn**., Calend.
  foamy; **Berb**.. **Carbo v.**. Cham.
  loose: Arn., Calend., Sil., Sul., Ustil.
  mouldy; Cham., Coch..
  shrivelled; Sul.
  slimy; Berb., *Camph*., **Carbo v.**, Sul.
  soft; Calc.p.
  sunken; Sul.
    with patches; Berb., Sul.
  thin; Calc.p.
  wet; Berb., Bov., Equis., Sil.
flabby: Sul.
straggly: Calc.p., Sil., Sul.
thin; Calc.p.
thrive; faliure to; Calc., Sil., Sul. Val.

Roots

damaged; Arn.
discolouration;
  red: Amm.c.
  whitish: Val.
dry; Amm.c., Berb., Sul.
exudate:
  frothy: Berb.
  viscid: Berb. Camph.
lumpy; Zinc m.
mouldy: Tromb.
pale: Vib.
short and brown: Calc.
slimy; Camph., Sil., Sul.
smell;
  bad; All.c.
  putrid; Bov.
swelling: Amm.c.
vesicles; Amm.c.,Sul. Val. Zinc m.
  red: Berb.
  white: Berb., Val.

Stems

bark;
  dry and harsh; Calc.fl.
chalky look; Calc.
rot; Calc.p.,
  base; Calc.fl.
  nodes; Calc.fl.
tillering;
  distorted; Calc.fl.
  numerous; Calc.fl., Calc.p.
  poor; Acon.,
  sterile; Calc.p.
lodging; Amm.m., Berb., Calc.p., Camph.
  from waterlogging: Camph.
swollen;
  base; Calc.p.
  nodes; Calc.f.
  oedematous; Samb.

Capillary

congestion; Acon., Samb., **Sul.**, Tromb.
disturbed; Sul., Urea.
engorged; Amm.c., Amm.m., Zinc m.
  sap decomposes; Amm.m., Sul.
  sap lost; Amm.c., Arn., Bell.
Thirst;
  diminished: Berb., Calend. Sil.
  frequent; Amm.c.
  increased; All.c., Amm.c., Amm.m., Berb., Bov., Calc., Camph., Sul., Val. Zinc m.
    afternoon and evening: Bov.
    but worse watering; Acon.

Leaves

blistering: Bell.
burn; Bell.
chalky look; Calc.
discolouration;
  chorosis: Acet. ac., Amm.c., Calc., Sil., Sul., Urea. Zinc m.
    Interveinal;
      pink; Calc., Sul.
      red: Bell.
      yellow-orange or pale yellow; Acon.
      yellow-brown with green edges and veins: Calc.
  crimson pink: Bell.
  mottling; Calc.
  purple; Sul.
  yellow; Calc.
    margins;
      red; Calc.
      yellow; Calc.p.
    tips;
      orange: Zinc m.
      red: Acon.
        afer injury; Arn.
      purple; Bell.
      yellow; Zinc m.
droopy; All.c.
dry: Calc.p.
evaporation;
  deficient; **Acet. ac**., *Acon*., All.c., Amm.carb., Cit.ac. Oxal.ac.
    night: Samb.
  excessive; **Acet. ac.,** *Berb.,* **Cit.ac., Oxal.ac**. Val. Vib.
    day; Samb.
  impaired; **Acet. ac.**, Acon., Amm.carb., Bell. Cit.ac., Oxal.ac. Tromb.

fall early; Amm.c., Bell.
hard; Sil.
leathery; Calc.p.
rolled; Calc.p.
unfurl;
  fail; Bell.
photosynthesis;
  impared; **Acet.ac.** All.c.**,** *Amm.c., Amm.m.,* Berb., **Camph., Cit.ac., Oxal.ac., Nat.sal. Sal.ac.** *Sul. Tromb., Urea., Val.* Vib.
respiration;
  deficient; **Acet.ac., Amm.c.,** *Berb.,* **Camph., Cit.ac., Oxal.ac.** *Tromb.*
rust;
  both sides of leaf; Amm.c.
  oval pustules: Amm.c.
spots; Tromb.
  red; Sil.
swellings; Bell., Calc.
  broad shiney; Acon.
  hard red; Acon., Arn.
wilting; Calc.
  rapid; Acon.
  slow; Camph.
  after transplanting; Arn., Calend.
wrinkled; Calc.p.

Flowers

collapse; calc.
  barley florets die; Calc.fl.
drooping; Kali c.
dry; Acon., Nat.c.
hot; Acon.
petals:
  absent; Cup.m. Ferr.s., Kali c., Nat.c.
  discoloured; Kali c.
  malformed; Bov., Cup.m. Ferr.s., Kali c., Nat.c. Teucr.
  pale; Sul.
premature; Amm.c., Bov., Calc., Nat.c. Sil., Sul., Val.
secretion;
  slimy: Amm.m.
shortlasting; Calc.
shrivelled; Bov., Cup.m. Ferr.s., Kali c., Nat.c.
small; Sil., Val.

Generative

ovaries
- immature; Berb., Bov., Cup.m. Ferr.s., Kali c., Nat.c.
- shrivelled; Bov., Kali c., Nat.c., Vib.
- sterility; Amm.c., Bov., Nat.c. Zinc m.

pollination; Ferr.m., Nat.c.
- absent; Amm.c., Berb., Bov., Cup.m., Nat.c. Ferr.s., Kali c.
- at night; Camph.
- defective; Bov., Cup.m., Ferr.s., Kali c., Nat.c. Sul.
- excessive; Acon., Amm.c., Calc.p., Ferr.m. Ruta.
- impared; Bov., Cup.m., Ferr.s., Kali c., Nat.c. Sil.
- premature; Zinc m.

stamen;
- excessive; Ferr.m.
- immature; Bov., Cup.m., Ferr.s., Kali c., Nat.c. Sil.
- long; Calc.p.
- shrivelled; Berb., Bov., Cup.m. Kali c., Nat.c.

Fruits

absent; Calc., Ferr.m., Ferr.s., Sul.
diminished; Amm.c., Berb., Calc., Ferr.m., Ferr.s., Kali c., Zinc m.
fall early; Bell., Calc., Sil., Vib.
red fruits look pale: Bell.
ripening;
- slow; Calc. Sil.

rotting; Ferr.p., Ferr.s., Calc.p.
- avocados; Calc.fl.
- brown rot; All.c.

set;
- poor: Camph., Ruta, Sil., Teuc.
- failure; Calc.
- slow; Acon.

skin;
- soft; Calc.p.

small; Bell., Calc., Calc.p.
spongey: Calc.
unhealthy; Calc., Ferr.m., Ferr.s.
- with blossom end rot; Ferr.s., Ocym.
- with maggots; Ferr.s.
- with caterpillars; Ferr.s.

Seed

absent; Calc., Sil., Sul.
seed bath: Sil
spongey; Calc.
sterile
  grain: Acon.
  fruit; Calc.

Named Diseases

anthracnose: *Arn.*, Bell., Calc., *Calend.*, **Carbo v., Nat.sal.**, Ocym., Phos., **Sal.ac.**, Sat.
bitterpip; Calc.
blight: All.c., Ferr.m., Ferr.p. Hyssop., Mang., Phos., Sul.
  early: All.c., Mang., Sul.
  halo; Nat.m., Nat.p., Phos., Sat., Sul.
  late: All.c., Sul.
  stripe; Nat.m., Nat.p., Phos., Sul.
  with:
    bacterium; Ferr.m., Ferr.p., Hyssop., Lact.ac., **Nat.sal.**, Ocym., Phos., **Sal.ac.**, Sat., Sul.
    fungus: Equis., Sil.
    nematode: **Calend.**, Calc.fl., Calc.p., Carbo v., Nast., **Tanac., Teuc.** Val.
    virus; **Acon., Bell.**, Kali m., **Nat.sal., Sal.ac.**
blotch; Calc.fl.. Calc.p., Mag.s., Mang., Nat.c., *Nit.ac.*, Phos., Sul.
  glume; Ferr.s., Mang., Nat.c., *Nit.ac.* Phos., Sul.
  septoria; Ferr.s., Mang., Nat.c., *Nit.ac.*, Phos., Sul.
damping off: Calc. C., **Carbo v.**, Cham., Mag.c., Mag.s.
dieback; Equis., *Sil.,* Ustil.
ergot; Kali s., Nat.sul., **Sec.** Ust.
  early stage: Amm.m.
gall; Sul., Thuja.
  crown; Sul.
  root; Sul.
gangrene; All.c., Lapis, **Nat.sal.**, Sil., **Sal.ac.,** Sul.
lather leaf: Sul.
mildew; Calc.p., Equis., Ferr.s., Kali m., Kali perm., Lact.ac., Mag.s., Mang., *Nit.ac.*, Sil., Sul.
  downy; All.c., Calc.p. Ferr.s., Kali m., Kali perm., Lact.ac., Mag.s. *Nit.ac.*, Sul.
  powdery; All.c., Equis., Ferr.s., Kali m., Sil. Kali perm., Lact. ac., Mag.s., *Nit.ac.*, Sul.
mould; Equis., Ferr.s., Kali m., Mang., **Nat.sal.**, Sil., Sul., **Sal.ac.**, Val.
  black; Ferr.s., Sul., Val.
  dry; Bov., Equis., Sil., **Nat.sal.**, Mang., Sul., Val.
  grey; Ferr.s., Kali m., Sul.

slimy; Val.
sooty; Calc.p., **Coccus., Shell.**
wet; Bov., **Nat.sal. Sal.ac.** Sul.
oedema; Berb., Sil.
rot; Berb., Bov., **Carbo v.** Equis., Hyssop., Phos., Sil. Sul.
armillaria root; Phos.
bacterial soft; Hyssop., Lact.ac., Nat.p., Phos., Sul.
bitter; Calend.
black; Lact.ac., Lapis
blossom end; Lapis
brown; All.c., Coch., Phos., Sul.
collar; Nat.p., Phos., Sul.
crown; Kali m., Sul.
dry; Berb., Bov., **Carbo v.** Coch., Equis., Lact.ac., Phos., Sil., Sul.
root; Phos.
soft; Lact.ac., Phos., Sul.
stem; Amm.m., Calc.fl., Calc.p.. Sul.
wet; Amm.m., Berb., Bov., **Carbo v.** Equis., Sil., Sul.
engorged; Berb.
foamy; **Nat.sal., Sal.ac.**, Sul.
slimy; Equis., Sil., **Nat.sal.**, Sul.
with patches; **Nat.sal.**, Sil., **Sal.ac**., Sul.
shrivelled; Equis., Sil., **Nat.sal.**, Sul.
rust (*puccinia* spp): Sul., Val.
banana; **Acon., Bell.** Canth.
bean; **Acon., Bell.** Canth., Sat.
chrysanthemum; **Acon**., Amm.carb., **Bell**. Canth.
iris; **Acon., Bell.** Canth.
leaf; **Acon., Amm.carb., Bell**. Berb., *Canth.*, Ferr.m., *Ferr.p.* Nat. sul., *Phos.*, Sat., Sul.
marigold; **Acon., Bell.**
pelargonium; **Acon.**, Amm.carb., **Bell.,** Canth.
poplar; **Acon., Bell.**
rose; **Acon., Bell.**
snapdragon; **Acon., Bell**.
stem; **Acon**., Amm.carb., **Bell.** Berb., Canth., Ferr.m., Nat.sul., Sat., Sul.
stripe; **Acon**., Amm.carb., **Bell**. Berb., Canth., Ferr.m., Nat.sul., Sul.
scab;
apple; All.c., Zinc.
citrus; Zinc.
head; Ustil. Zinc.
potato; Ustil. Zinc.
powdery; All.c., Zinc.
rhizoctonia; Zinc.
violet; Zinc.
scald; Nat.m., Ocym., Phos.
smut; Ustil.

bunt; Ustil.
flag; Ustil.
loose; Ustil.
speck;
grey; Kali perm.
spot;
angular leafspot; Sat.
black; Ferr.m., Ferr.p. *Nit.ac.,* Sat., Sul.
brown; Sat.
eye; Nat.c., Sul.
halo; Nat.sul., **Samb.,** Sul.
leafspot; Sat.
stripe;
bacterial; Ferr.m., Ferr.p., **Nat.sal. Sal.ac.**
black; Nat.sul., Sul.
halo; Phos.
rust; **Acon.**, Amm.carb., **Bell.**, *Canth.*
take-all; Mang.
virus;
alfalfa virus; **Nat.sal., Sal.ac.**
barley yellow dwarf; **Acon., Bell.,** Kali m., **Nat.sal., Sal.ac**.
mosaic; Lact.ac., Lapis, **Nat.sal., Sal.ac.**
potato virus; **Nat.sal. Sal.ac.**
tobacco mosaic virus; Lact.ac., Lapis, **Nat.sal.** Ocym., **Sal.ac.**
wilt;
fusarium wilt; Ocym., Sat.
spotted wilt; Ocym., Sat.
windrowing: **Carbo v.**, Mag.c., Nat.c.

Pests

General: Acon., All.c., Amm.c., Aran., Bell., **Bombyx.**, *Car.*, **Coccin. Chrysop**., Hyssop. Kali c., Men., Nast., **Nat.sal.**, Nat.sul., Ocym., Ricin., **Ruta., Sal.ac.**, Salvia., *Samb*., Sat., Sil., **Staphyl., Syrph., Tanac., Teuc.,** Thuja. Vib.
acacia spotting bug; Bell.
ants; Camph., **Calend**., Men., **Tanac. Teuc**.
white; camph.
aphids; All.c. Amm.c., **Coccin**., Chrysop., Men., Nast., Nat.c., **Nat.sal.** Nat.sul., Ocym., Phos., **Sal.ac.**. Salvia., Samb., Sil., Syrph.
with yellow dwarf virus; **Acon., Bell**., **Nat.sal.,** Ocym., Phos., **Sal. ac.**
beetles; **Aran**. Calend., Canth., Hyssop. Men., Ocym., Phos., Sat., Sil., **Staphyl**. Thuja.
asparagus; Calend.
bean beetle; Sat., **Staphyl., Syrph.**
blister beetle; Camph., Canth., **Staphyl., Syrph.**
flea beetle; Hyssop.

fruit; Phos., Sil.
japanese; *Tanac.*
bugs; Aran. Canth., Ferr.m., Hyssop. Kali c., Kali perm., Nast., Ocym., Sat., Staphyl., Sul., Thuja.
bronze orange; Camph., Canth.
fruit spotting; Phos., Sul.
mealy; Nast., **Staphyl., Syrph**.
sow; **Porc.**
squash; Nast., **Staphyl., Syrph**.
caterpillars; **Bombyx**., **Car., Coccin**., Hyssop., Men., Nat. c., *Ocym*., Ricin., Salvia., **Samb**., Sat., Sil., **Staphyl**., Sul., **Syrph., Tanac., Teuc.**, *Thuja*., Val., Vib.
army worms; All.c., *Bombyx*., **Car., Samb., Staphyl., Syrph.**, *Tanac.*
budworm; All.c., *Bombyx*., *Car*., **Samb., Sil., Staphyl., Syrph.,** *Tanac.*
cabbage moth; All.c., **Aran.,** *Bombyx.,* **Car.,** Hyssop., Salv., **Staphyl., Syrph**., *Tanac.*
cluster caterpillar; Aran., **Bombyx., Car., Samb., Staphyl., Syrph.,** Tanac.
cutworm; All.c., *Bombyx*., *Car*., **Samb., Staphyl., Syrph.,** *Tanac.*
loopers; All.c., *Bombyx*., *Car*., **Staphyl., Syrph.,** *Tanac.*
procession moth; All.c., **Aran., Bombyx., Car., Staphyl., Syrph.,** *Tanac.*
sawfly larvae; All.c., Aran., **Bombyx., Car., Staphyl., Syrph.,** Tanac.
spitfire; **Aran., Bombyx., Car., Samb., Staphyl., Syrph.,** *Tanac.*
webworm; **Aran., Bombyx., Car., Samb., Staphyl., Syrph.,** *Tanac.*
cockroaches; All.c., Aran., Camph.
crickets; Aran. Hyssop. Staphyl.
flies; All.c. Aran. **Bombyx**., Hyssop., Nast., Ocym., **Ruta**., Salvia., Samb. Sat., **Staphyl., Syrph., Tanac., Teuc.**, Tromb., Thuja.
blow: Tromb.
cabbage fly; *Tanac., Teuc.*
carrotfly; All.c., Aran., Salv.
fruitfly; Ocym., Phos., Sul.
gnat; Hyssop.
onion fly; All. c.
sawfly; All.c., Aran., **Bombyx**., Hyssop., Ocym., Salvia., **Samb**. Sat., Sil., **Staphylinida, Syrph., Tanac.,** Thuja., Val., Vib.
stable: Tromb.
katydids; Aran., Hyssop., Ocym., Sat., Thuja.
leafhoppers; Kali perm., Ocym., **Staphylinida., Syrph**.
leafminers; Ocym., Sat., Thuja.
maggots; Aran., Delia., Hyssop., Ocym., Sat., **Staphylinida, Syrph**., Thuja.
mites; **Acon**., All.c. Bell., **Bov**., **Coccin**., Mag.p., Nat.c., Ocym., Ricin., Salvia., Sil., Sul., **Tromb**., Thuja., Val., Vib.
blister mite; **Coccin.**, Thuja. Sul.
citrus mite: Sil.
redlegged mite; **Coccin**., Lact.ac., Ocym.
russet mite; **Coccin**., Ocym.
rust mite; Acon., **Aran.,** Bell., **Bombyx., Car**., Ricin., **Staphyl., Syrph**., Thuja.

spidermite; **Coccin**., Bov., Lact.ac., Tromb
tomato; **Coccin**. Ocym.
two-spotted mite; **Coccin**., Ocym., Sul.
vinemite; Ricin., Salv.
mosquitos; **Coccin.,** Ocym.
moths; Aran. **Bombyx**., *Camph*., Hyssop., Men., Ocym., Ricin., Salvia., **Samb**. Sat., Sil., Staphyl., Sul., **Tanac., Teuc.**, Thuja., Val., Vib.
cabbage moth; All.c., **Aran**., Bombyx., **Car**., Hyssop., **Staphylinida., Syrph., Tanac.**
diamondback; **Aran., Bombyx., Car., Coccin. Samb., Staphylinida., Syrph., Tanac.**
fruit moth; Aran., Bombyx., Caribida., Phos., Staphylinida., Syrph.
grapevine moth; **Aran., Bombyx., Car.**, Ricin., **Staphylinida., Syrph., Tanac.**
hawk moth; **Aran., Bombyx., Car.,** Ricin., **Staphylinida., Syrph.**, Thuja.
potato moth; **Aran., Bombyx., Car., Samb., Staphylinida., Syrph., Tanac.**
procession moth; All.c., **Aran., Bombyx., Car., Staphylinida., Syrph., Tanac.**
nematodes; **Calend**., Calc.fl., Calc.p., *Carbo v.,* Nast., Sul., **Tanac., Teuc.,** Val., Zinc m.
root knot; **Calend.,** Sul.**, Tanac., Teuc.,** Val. Zinc m.
sawfly; All.c., Aran., **Bombyx**., Hyssop., Ocym., Salvia., **Samb**. Sat., Sil. **Staphylinida., Syrph., Tanac.**
scales; All. c., **Coccin., Coccus.,** Salvia.**, Shellac.** Thuja.
hard; **Bombyx.**, Car., **Coccin**., Salvia., **Shellac.**
honeydew; **Coccus., Shellac.**
soft; **Bombyx.**, Car., **Coccin**., Salvia., **Shellac.**
slater: **Nat. Sal., Porcell., sal. ac**.
snails; Helix. Kali perm.
termites; **Camph.**
thrips; **Acon**., All.c., **Aran**., Bell., Calc.c., **Car.**, Hyssop., Kali s., Nat.sul., *Ocym*., Phos., Sat., **Staphylinida., Syrph.**, *Thuja.*, *Val.*
bean bossom thrips: **Acon**., Val.
banana rust thrips: Amm.c., Bell., Val.
vermin; All.c.
wasps; **Aran**., Hyssop., Sat., **Staphylinida., Syrph.**, Thuja.
weevils; All.c., **Aran**., Ferr.s., Hyssop., Nat.c., Ocym., Sat., **Staphylinida.**, Thuja.
woodworm: **Camph.**

Nutrients

crave**; All.c.**
nutrient deficiency**;**
ammonium: Amm. c., Kali nit.
boron: Borax.
calcium: **Ferr., Mag., Mang., Phos., Sul., Zinc.**
carbon: **Sil.**
copper: **Ferr., Molyb., Phos.**, *Sil.*, **Sul., Zinc**.

iron: **Cup.m., Kali., Mang., Phos., Zinc.**
magnesium: **Calc.c., Kali., Nat., Phos.,** Sul.
manganese: **Calc.c., Ferr., Kali., Mag., Phos.**
molybdenum: *Amm.c.*, **Cup.m.,** *Kali.n., Nit.ac.,* **Phos., Sul.**
nitrogen: Molyb.
phosphorus: **Alum., Calc.c., Ferr.,** *Kali.nit.*, **Mag., Mang., Nat.m., Zinc.**
potassium: **Ferr., Mang., Nat.m.**, Sul.
silica; **Carbo.v.**
sodium; Sul.
sulphur: **Calc.c., Cup.m.,** Kali.nit., **Molyb., Zinc.**
zinc: **Ferr., Calc.c., Cup.m., Phos., Sul.**

nutrient excess:
boron: Borax.
calcium: **Ferr., Mag., Mang., Phos., Sul. Zinc.**
carbon: **Sil.**
copper: **Ferr., Molyb., Phos.,** *Sil.*, **Sul., Zinc.**
iron: **Cup.m., Kali., Mang., Phos., Zinc.**
magnesium: **Calc.c., Kali., Nat., Phos.**
manganese: **Calc.c., Ferr., Kali., Mag., Phos. Sil.**
molybdenum: *Amm.c.*, **Cup.m.,** *Kali.n., Nit.ac.,* **Phos., Sul.**
nitrogen: Calc., *Molyb.*
phosphorus: **Alum., Calc.c., Ferr., Mag., Mang., Nat.m., Zinc.**
potassium: **Ferr., Mang., Nat.m.**
silica; **Carbo.v.**
sulphur: **Calc.c., Cup.m., Molyb., Zinc.**
zinc: **Ferr., Calc.c., Cup.m., Phos., Sul.**

poor uptake: **All.c.,** Sil., Sul., Tromb., Vib.

Cause

bacterial; **Nat.sal. Sal.ac.**
disease; Acet.ac.. **Acon.**, Amm.c., **Bell.**, *Cit.ac.*, Ferr.m., Ferr.p., Nat.c., *Oxal.ac.*
fertiliser; **Amm.carb., Nit.ac., Kali.nit.**
fungal; Berb., Bov., **Carbo v.** Coch., Equis., Sil.
heavy metal poisoning; Sul.
herbicide: Sul.
injury; **Arn., Calend.**,Carbo v., **Cham.**, Ferr.p. Sil.
fire; Acon., Bell., Canth., Caps., **Carbo v.**, Ferr.m., Ferr.p., **Nat.sal. Sal. ac.**, Sul.
insect; **Acon.**, *All.c., Amm.c., Aran.*, **Bell., Bombyx.**, *Car.*, **Coccin.** Chrysop., Ferr. s., Hyssop., Kali nit., Kali perm., Men., Nast., Nat. sal., Ocym., Ricin., **Ruta.**, Sal. ac., Salvia., Samb., Sat., Staphyl., Syrph., **Tanac., Teuc.,** Thuja, Val.
mechanical; Acon., **Arn., Calend., Carbo v**. Ferr.m., Ferr.p.
open wounds and lacerations; Calend.

nematodes; Calend.
transplants; Calend., Sil.
grafts/cuttings; Calend., Sil.
storm; **Arn., Calend., Carbo v.**, Ferr. m., Ferr. p., **Nat. sal., Sal. ac.**
sunburn; Acon., Bell., Carbo v., **Canth., Caps.**
windrowing; **Carbo v.**, nat sul., Sul.
nematode; **Calend**., Nast., **Tanac., Teuc**. Val.
salination;
bores; Mag.s., Nat.m.
fertiliser run-off; Mag.p., Mag.s., Nat.c., Nat.m., Nat.sul.
natural salts; Mag.p., Mag.s., Nat.c., Nat.m., Nat.sul.
viral; **Acon**., Amm., **Bell**. *Canth.*, **Nat.sal. Sal.ac.**
waterlogging;
drainage; Val.
salination; Mag.p., Mag.s., Nat.c., Nat.m., Nat.sul.

Modalities

worse;
light: Acon., Bell.
manuring: Tromb.
night: Sul.
watering; Acon., Tromb.
weather;
cloudy: Zinc m.
cold dry nights: Acon.
cold air; Amm.c., Amm.m., Calc., Calc.p., Camph., Tromb.
heat: Sul.
warm to cold; Bell.
wet; Amm.c., Amm.m., Calc.p., Camph., *Sul.* Zinc m.
wind: Bell., Sul.
stormy; Amm.c.
better;
warmth: Amm.c., Calc.
wind; Val.
speed:
rapid; Acon., Bell.

Future Development

Compared with the hundreds of years of cooperative international research between thousands of homoeopaths focused upon human health, the work presented here is paltry. Whilst I hope that it is clear that what has been presented is a reasonable foundation, it is equally clear that so much more needs to be done to reveal the potential of the discipline.

One would like the idea to catch on sufficiently so that people are motivated to make experiments with all sorts of crops and remedies in all parts of the world. Even as research, this is approachable by individuals with single crops in their gardens just as much as research faculties with all the equipment and expertise honed on more aggressive technologies. Such research would, ideally, be collated and the democratic process of science brought to bear upon it; discussion, peer review, the elucidation of the underlying concepts, the reinforcement of good research and the adaptation of lesser findings. Perhaps it will be successful and we can all be part of the development of a cheap and non-toxic agriculture. It's not such a bad dream I think.

To facilitate this vision, in cooperation with the publisher, a web site investigating biodynamic agriculture has been adapted to try to realise this future - or one with similar aims.

The site can be found at **http://www.considera.org**. Follow the link to 'preparations' and you will find the work presented in this book augmented by a fuller repertory structure and compatible remedies from other disciplines and research.

The suggestions I have made in this book do not dominate the site. If classical homoeopathic principles and practice is appropriate (as I strongly believe), then this will emerge through its own strengths. If not ... perhaps there will be something to bring back to homoeopathy for people and veterinary physicians.

My contribution is now out in the world and, in the end, 'by their fruits shall ye know them'.

Bibliography

Books

Materia Medica of the Guiding Symptoms with Keynotes. Boericke W. 1923 USA Reprint B. Jain 1990 India.
Dictionary of Practical Materia Medica. Clarke J.H. 1900 UK Reprint B. Jain 1991 India.
Treatise on Micro-immunotherapy Julian O.A. 1982 France Reprint B.Jain 1989 India.
The Bio-chemic System of Medicine Schuessler W 1888 Germany Reprint B.Jain 1984 India.
The Homoeopathic Materia Medica Teste A 1853 France Reprint B.Jain 1992 India
The Guiding Symptoms of our Materia Medica Hering C. 1848 USA Reprint B.Jain 1992 India
Encyclopedia of Materia Medica Allen T.F. 1863 USA Reprint B.Jain 1992 India
Materia Medica Pura Hahnemann S. 1790 Germany Reprint B.Jain 1984 India.
The Chronic Diseases Hahnemann S. 1834 Germany Reprint B.Jain 1984 India
Organon of Medicine Hahnemann S 1843 France Reprint B. Jain 1990 India
Forty Years Practise Jahr 1855 Germany Reprint B.Jain 1936 India
Leaders in Homoeopathic Therapeutics Nash E.B. 1890 UK Reprint B.Jain 1942 India
Textbook of Homoeopathic Materia Medica Leeser O. 1932 Germany Reprint B.Jain 1983 India
A Modern Herbal Grieve M.A. 1931 UK Reprint Dover Publications 1964 USA
Medicinal Plants Millspaugh C.F. 1892 USA Yorston USA
Hemphill's Book of Herbs Hemphill J. & R. 1991 Australia Child and associates Australia.
The Rodale Herbbook Hylton W. H. Editor 1974 USA Rodale Press USA
Herbal Handbook For Farm and Stable. de Bairachi Levy J. 1952 UK Reprint Rodale press 1976 USA
Companion Plants Philbrick H. and Gregg B. 1966 USA Reprint Robinson and Watkins 1972 UK
Pests Predators and Pesticides Conacher J. 1979 Australia Reprint Organic growers ass. 1991 Australia
General Botany Fuller H.J. and Ritchie D.D. 1941 USA Reprint Harper and Row 1967 USA
The Plant Kingdom Tribe I. 1970 UK Hamlin UK
Comparative Examinations of Plants Suffering from Potash Deficiency. Bussler W. 1962 Germany Reprint Verlag Chemie Germany
What Garden Pest or Disease is That? McMaugh J. 1986 Australia Landsdown Publishing 1995 Australia
Biological Pestcontrol Hussey N.W. and Scopes N.E.A. 1985 UK Blandford Press UK

Chemistry of Organic Medical Products. Jenkins G.L. Hastung W.H. 1949 USA John Wing and Sons Inc. USA
Department of Agriculture WA Farmnotes: Symptoms of Nutrient Deficiencies in Rape Farmnote (No number) Agdex (no number) Mason and Gartrell (undated)
Nitrogen and Phosphorus Disorders of Vegetable Crops McPharlin I and Phillips D. 1989 Bulletin no 4175 Agdex no 250/236
Causes of Fruitdrop Whiteley K.T. 1983 Farmnote 71/83 Agdex 210/20
Trace Elements and Magnesium Treatments for Apple and Pear Trees Shorter N.H. and Cripps J.E.L. 1985 Farmnote 45/85 Agdex 211/541
Molybdenum Deficiencies in Vegetables Floyd R. 1986 Farmnote 88/86 Agdex 250/632

Periodicals

Effect of Copper Application on Take-All Severity and Grass yield of Wheat Brennan R.F. 1991 Australian journal of experimental agriculture 31/255-8
Effect of Additions of Nitrogen and Sulphur to Irrigated Wheat at Heading Randall et al. 1990 Australian journal of experimental agriculture 30/95-101
Potassium Nutrition of Irrigated Potatoes in South Australia Maier N.A. et al. 1989 Australian journal of experimental agriculture 29/419-32
Implications of Soiltype, Pasture Composition and Mineral Content Lewis D.C. and Sparrow L.A. 1991 Australian journal of experimental agriculture 31/609-15
Diagnostic Indices for Sulphur Status of Subterranean Clover. Spencer K et al. 1977 Australian Journal of Agricultural Research. 28/401-12
Effects of Previous Superphosphate Applications on Pasture McLachlan K.D. and Norman B.W. 1962 Australian Journal of Agricultural Research. 13/5 832-52
Nitrogen Use of Trickle Irrigated Tomatoes Stark et al. 1983 Agronomy journal 75/672-6
Improved Nitrogen Management in Irrigated Durum Wheat Knowles et al. 1991 Agronomy journal 83/346-52
Influence of Mycorrhizal Fungi on Mineral Nutrition Ojala J.C. et al. 1983 Agronomy journal 75/255-9
Nitrogen Sources Effects on Rabbit-eye Blueberry Plant and Soil Interaction Patten et al. 1988 Communications in soil science and plant analysis 19/1065-74
Virus Infection and Nutrient Elemental Content of the Host Plant Kaplan R.C. and Gergman E.L. 1985 Communications in soil science and plant analysis 16/439-65
Growth and Tissue Composition of Sweet Corn as Affected by Nitrogen Source Rudert B.D. and Locascio S.J. 1979 Journal of the American Society of Horticultural Science 104 /520-3
The Effect of Chlorsulfuron on the Uptake of Copper and Zinc in Wheat. Robson A.D. and Snowball K. 1990 Journal of the American Society of Horticultural Science 118/526-32

Nitrate Monitoring for Pumpkin Production on Dry Land and Irrigated Soils Swaider J.M. et al. 1988 Journal of the American Society of Horticultural Science 113/684-9

Plant Analysis, an Interpretation Manual. Robson A.D. Snowball K. 1986 Inkata Press Australia

Effect of super and Nitrogen on Take-all and Yield of Wheat Brennan R.F. 1992 Fertiliser Research 31/43-49

The Role of Manganese and Nitrogen in Susceptibility of Wheat to Take-all Brennan R.F. 1992 Fertiliser research 31 /35-41

Interactions Between Nutrients in Higher Plants. Robson A.D. Pitman M.G. 1983 Springer Verlag Germany

Some Chemical Properties of Soils from Areas of Barleygrass Infestation Nelson A.J. et al. 1971 New Zealand journal of agricultural research 14/334-51

Cultural Innovation: its Implications for Mushroom Pestcontrol Hussey N.W. 1981 The Congress Australia.

Effect of Salvia on Growth of Grass. Muller C.H. & W.H. Haines B.L. 1964 Science Newsletter UCA USA

Soil and Plant Analysis Special Edition 1993 CSIRO Australia

Fertilisation Management of Crops Irrigated with Saline Water. Feigin A. 1985 Plant and Soil 89/285-99

Nitrogen Fertilisation under Saline Conditions in Tomatoes and Cucumbers Cerda A. Martinez V. 1988 Journal of horticultural science 63/451-8

Photo Credits

p35	t	© Bettmann/CORBIS
p36	t	© Lindsay Hebberd/CORBIS
	b	© ANNEBICQUE BERNARD/CORBIS SYGMA
p37	t-l	Green peach aphid Scott Bauer, USDA Agricultural Research Service*
	t-r	Cabbage aphid infestation Whitney Cranshaw, Colorado State University*
	b	Sevenspotted lady beetle Russ Ottens, The University of Georgia*
p38	t	Keeled slug Boris Hrasovec, University of Zagreb*
	m	Monacha cartusiana Luboš Kolouch*
	b	Spanish slugs Luboš Kolouch*
p39	t-r	©Ian Britton/Freefoto.com
	b-r	BdMax New Zealand
p40	b-r	Orb weaver adult Joseph Berger*
p41	t-l	St. John's wart midge Norman E. Rees, USDA Agricultural Research Service*
	t-r	Goldenrod gall fly USDA Forest Service Ogden Archives*
	m-l	Sweetpotato weevil adult Clemson University USDA Cooperative Extension Slide Series *
	u-m-r	Carrot weevil adult Alton N. Sparks, Jr., The University of Georgia*
	l-m-r	Apple scab damage Clemson University USDA Cooperative Extension Slide Series*
	b-r	Anthracnose on lima bean Clemson University USDA Cooperative Extension Slide Series*
p42	b-r	Stem nematode on garden onion Central Science Laboratory, Harpenden Archives, British Crown*
	b-l	Root-knot nematode on tobacco R.J. Reynolds Tobacco Company Slide Set, R.J. Reynolds Tobacco Company*
	c	Wheat seed-gall nematode Michael McClure, University of Arizona*
	m-l	Wheat seed-gall nematode G. Caubel, Institut National de la Recherche Agronomique*
	t-l	Root-knot nematode on rice Roger Lopez-Chaves, Universidad de Costa Rica*
	t-r	Wheat seed-gall nematode Jonathan D. Eisenback, Virginia Polytechnic Institute and State University*
P139	t	Damping off/Fusarium root rot in European beech Andrej Kunca, National Forest Centre Slovakia*
	b-l	Damping off/Fusarium root rot in silver fir Andrej Kunca, National Forest Centre Slovakia*
	b-r	Root rot/damping off tobacco Clemson University USDA Cooperative Extension Slide Series*
p140	t-l	Brown spot on tobacco R.J. Reynolds Tobacco Company Slide Set, R.J. Reynolds Tobacco Company*
	t-r	Eye spot on red maple Joseph O'Brien, USDA Forest Service*
	u-m-l	Strawberry leaf spot Clemson University USDA Cooperative Extension Slide Series*
	u-m-r	Black spot invades cabbage leaves Clemson University USDA Cooperative Extension Slide Series*
	l-m-l	Raspberry rust Courtesy of Minnesota Extension Service. www.extension.umn.edu
	b-r	Septoria leaf spot of wheat Clemson University USDA Cooperative Extension Slide Series*
	b-l	Oak anthracnose damage USDA Forest Service Archives, USDA Forest Service*
p141	t-l	Bacterial leaf scorch Theodor D. Leininger, USDA Forest Service*
	t-r	Bacterial blight on soyabean ENSA-Montpellier Archives, Ecole nationale suprieure agronomique de Montpellier*
	m-l	Anthracnose on ash Courtesy of Minnesota Extension Service. www.extension.umn.edu
	m-r	Downy mildew on melon Clemson University USDA Cooperative Extension Slide Series*
	b-l	Southern Bacterial Wilt / Potato Brown Rot leaf scorching Jean L. Williams-Woodward, The University of Georgia*
	b-r	Poplar/aspen rust Arthur L. Schipper, USDA Forest Service*
p142	t-l	Bean rust on snap bean Clemson University USDA Cooperative Extension Slide Series*
	t-r	Drowning burley tobacco R.J. Reynolds Tobacco Company Slide Set, R.J. Reynolds Tobacco Company*
	m-l	Powdery mildew on oak Clemson University USDA Cooperative Extension Slide Series*
	m-r	Tobacco mosaic virus R.J. Reynolds Tobacco Company Slide Set, R.J. Reynolds Tobacco Company*
	b-l	Fusarium wilt Clemson University - USDA Cooperative Extension Slide Series*
	b-r	Helminthosporium leaf blotch on oat Clemson University USDA Cooperative Extension Slide Series*
p143	t-l	Gray mold on strawberry Clemson University USDA Cooperative Extension Slide Series*
	t-r	Wheat seed-gall nematode Jonathan D. Eisenback, Virginia Polytechnic Institute and State University*
	b-l	Loose smut of wheat or barley Clemson University - USDA Cooperative Extension Slide Series*
	b-r	Corn smut Clemson University USDA Cooperative Extension Slide Series*
p144	t-r	Tobacco budworm R.J. Reynolds Tobacco Company Slide Set, R.J. Reynolds Tobacco Company*
	c-l	Squash bug on watermelon Alton N. Sparks, Jr., The University of Georgia*
	c-r	Twospotted spider mite on cotton Mississippi State University Archives, Mississippi State University*
	b-l	Asparagus beetle Clemson University USDA Cooperative Extension Slide Series*
	b-r	Diamondback moth pupae on cabbage Alton N. Sparks, Jr., The University of Georgia*
p145	t-l	Black dot spurge flea beetle on soft spurge USDA APHIS PPQ Archives*
	u-m-l	Mango seed weevil USDA APHIS PPQ Archives*
	l-m-l	Saddleback caterpillar Herbert A. "Joe" Pase III, Texas Forest Service*
	t-r	Aspen leafminer USDA Forest Service Ogden Archives*
	b-l	Diamondback moth larva Alton N. Sparks, Jr., The University of Georgia*
	b-r	Eriophyid mite on poplar/aspen Whitney Cranshaw, Colorado State University*

* Images sourced using www.forestryimages.org The publisher would like to express gratitude for this superb service and the generosity of those with whom there was correspondence.

All other images - Mark Moodie Publications.

Index

C

D

E

F

G

H

I

J

K

L

M

N

O

P

R

S

T

U

V

W

X

Y

Z

Dedication

To Pym, who was the first homoeopath to change my life, Dr. Chatterjee, who was my teacher, Silke Bauer, who prompted me to use remedies on plants, and to Alena Tetreault, who was instrumental in the completion of the book.